RECENT ADVANCES IN HEMATOLOGY RESEARCH

ERYTHROCYTES

STRUCTURE, FUNCTIONS AND CLINICAL ASPECTS

RECENT ADVANCES IN HEMATOLOGY RESEARCH

Additional books and e-books in this series can be found on Nova's website under the Series tab.

Recent Advances in Hematology Research

Erythrocytes

Structure, Functions and Clinical Aspects

Katy Jorissen
Editor

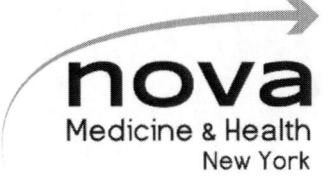
Medicine & Health
New York

Copyright © 2019 by Nova Science Publishers, Inc.

All rights reserved. No part of this book may be reproduced, stored in a retrieval system or transmitted in any form or by any means: electronic, electrostatic, magnetic, tape, mechanical photocopying, recording or otherwise without the written permission of the Publisher.

We have partnered with Copyright Clearance Center to make it easy for you to obtain permissions to reuse content from this publication. Simply navigate to this publication's page on Nova's website and locate the "Get Permission" button below the title description. This button is linked directly to the title's permission page on copyright.com. Alternatively, you can visit copyright.com and search by title, ISBN, or ISSN.

For further questions about using the service on copyright.com, please contact:
Copyright Clearance Center
Phone: +1-(978) 750-8400   Fax: +1-(978) 750-4470   E-mail: info@copyright.com.

NOTICE TO THE READER

The Publisher has taken reasonable care in the preparation of this book, but makes no expressed or implied warranty of any kind and assumes no responsibility for any errors or omissions. No liability is assumed for incidental or consequential damages in connection with or arising out of information contained in this book. The Publisher shall not be liable for any special, consequential, or exemplary damages resulting, in whole or in part, from the readers' use of, or reliance upon, this material. Any parts of this book based on government reports are so indicated and copyright is claimed for those parts to the extent applicable to compilations of such works.

Independent verification should be sought for any data, advice or recommendations contained in this book. In addition, no responsibility is assumed by the Publisher for any injury and/or damage to persons or property arising from any methods, products, instructions, ideas or otherwise contained in this publication.

This publication is designed to provide accurate and authoritative information with regard to the subject matter covered herein. It is sold with the clear understanding that the Publisher is not engaged in rendering legal or any other professional services. If legal or any other expert assistance is required, the services of a competent person should be sought. FROM A DECLARATION OF PARTICIPANTS JOINTLY ADOPTED BY A COMMITTEE OF THE AMERICAN BAR ASSOCIATION AND A COMMITTEE OF PUBLISHERS.

Additional color graphics may be available in the e-book version of this book.

Library of Congress Cataloging-in-Publication Data

ISBN: 978-1-53615-914-1

Published by Nova Science Publishers, Inc. † New York

Contents

Preface		vii
Chapter 1	Research Advances in Erythroid Development from Human Pluripotent Stem Cells *Yijin Chen, Bin Mao, Jia Feng, Yonggang Zhang and Feng Ma*	1
Chapter 2	Erythrocyte Disorders: Causes and Clinical Outcomes *R. Vani and R. Soumya*	21
Chapter 3	Erythrocyte Membranes: Unique Constituent of Biological/Hybrid Drug Delivery Systems *Ivana T. Drvenica, Ana Z. Stančić, Branko M. Bugarski, Ivana Pajic-Lijaković, Irina Maslovarić and Vesna Lj. Ilić*	57
Chapter 4	Electrochemical Properties of Erythrocytes as a Reflection of Their Morphology and Interaction with Foreign Electrically Conductive Materials *Mark M. Goldin, I. V. Goroncharovskaya, A. K. Evseev, A. K. Shabanov, Michael M. Goldin and S. S. Petrikov*	133
Index		161
Related Nova Publications		165

PREFACE

In Erythrocytes: Structure, Functions and Clinical Aspects, the authors summarize advances in human pluripotent stem cells-derived erythroid development and molecular regulatory mechanisms. This research may provide a new perspective on human embryo erythropoiesis and a possible treatment for some hematological diseases.

Erythrocytes are well equipped to carry out their functions due to a dynamic cell membrane, their inherent shape and lack of organelles and cytoplasmic viscosity. As such, the following section focusses on the causes of these modifications and their clinical implications.

As an example of complexity in research towards the development of erythrocyte membrane-based drug delivery systems starting from animal erythrocyte, morphological, biochemical and drug release profiles will be reviewed in the penultimate chapter.

The final chapter investigates the electrochemical behavior of erythrocytes at platinum, carbonaceous, and optically transparent electrodes via polarization and coulometric measurements. The order of magnitude of the quantity of electrons transferred between erythrocytes and electrodes was determined, and potential ranges showing indifference of the electrode toward red blood cells were identified.

Chapter 1 - Erythroid cells play an essential role in whole life of mammals, particularly in supporting the growth and survival of the embryo/fetus. Human erythropoiesis has already been precisely described in adult but not yet in embryo. Human pluripotent stem cells (hPSCs) are of great potential for tissue substitutes (for example, blood cells) and to cure various congenital disorders. So far, many laboratories have reported that mature erythrocytes could be efficiently generated from hPSCs using different methods. Recent reports show that hPSC-derived hematopoiesis follows two different pathways, and erythrocytes as the earliest developed blood cells have a unique developmental pathway through hematopoiesis. In this chapter, we summarize advances in hPSC-derived erythroid development and molecular regulatory mechanism. These researches may provide a new perspective on human embryo erythropoiesis and a possible treatment for some hematological diseases. The critical problems need to be solved and the research prospects of this field will also be addressed at the end of the chapter.

Chapter 2 - Erythrocytes or red blood cells (RBCs) are important constituents of blood, whose main function is to transport oxygen to tissues through hemoglobin. These cells are produced by erythropoiesis, mature in 8 days and have a life span of 120 days. Erythrocytes are enucleate, possess a specialized cell membrane and depend on glycolysis and pentose phosphate pathways for energy. Erythrocytes are well equipped to carry out their functions due to a dynamic cell membrane, their inherent shape & lack of organelles and cytoplasmic viscosity. Alterations in their structure and properties cause impairments in functioning and reduce survival. This chapter focusses on the causes of these modifications and their clinical implications. Erythrocyte disorders can be broadly divided into the following categories:

1. Membrane disorders: Variations in the structure of the membrane and shape of RBCs can be due to:
   - Skeletal defects reduce mechanical resistance and lifespan (hereditary spherocytosis, hereditary elliptosis, hereditary pyropoikilocytosis and South Asian ovalocytosis)
   - Changes in cation permeability and transport reduces osmotic resistance (hereditary stomatocytosis)
   - Other causes - oxidative stress and increase in calcium levels

2. Hemoglobinopathies: Disorders due to globin gene mutations such as sickle cell disease and thalassemia also cause secondary effects.
3. Volume homeostasis:
   - Primary disorders include inherent disorders of volume regulation (hereditary xerocytosis)
   - Secondary diseases due to other RBC disorders
4. Oxidative stress:
   - Production of reactive species in RBCs, which directly leads to protein oxidation and lipid peroxidation
   - Other acute and chronic diseases such as cardiovascular diseases, malaria, liver disease, etc.
5. Metabolic disorders or Enzymopathies: Defects in enzymes related to:
   - Glycolysis - pyruvate kinase, hexokinase, aldolase, etc.
   - Hexose monophosphate shunt - glucose-6-phosphate dehydrogenase, glutathione peroxidase, etc.
   - Other enzyme deficiencies - pyrimidine-5'-nucleotidase, ATPase, etc.

These disorders, either as primary causes or in association with other conditions, clinically manifest into anemia and its related ailments. Anemia is triggered by blood loss, surge in erythrocyte destruction or impairment in their production and also by variations in erythrocyte shape, size and hemoglobin content. Supplementation of iron, folic acid and vitamin B_{12} are used to treat mild cases of anemia, while RBC transfusions are preferred in severe cases. Transfusions are the primary interventions employed to subside the severity of erythrocyte disorders. Better blood banking and increased availability of blood would provide far reaching effects into the treatment of erythrocyte disorders.

Chapter 3 - For many decades, the red blood cell membranes were in focus of research interest solely as a model system for investigation into the various membrane-related phenomena, composition/organization or membrane transport properties, as well as the comparative proteomic and lipidomic analyses in health and disease. During 50s, along with the first experimental steps in ATP encapsulation in erythrocytes membranes, these entities begin to fascinate clinicians and researchers by their super carrier capabilities for the controlled and targeted delivery (vascular, pulmonary, subcutaneous) of wide range of conventional drugs and biologicals. A relatively new realm for erythrocyte membrane is its application in targeted delivery of nanoparticles, like erythrocyte membrane cloaked nanoparticles, incorporating their most useful traits such as long circulation and stealth features. This chapter focuses on red blood cell membrane as unique constituent of drug delivery systems, including nano-sized ones (nanoerythrosomes) and *ex vivo* technologies for their preparation. Rheological characterization of membranes as well as the change induced by various experimental conditions is prerequisite for their application as drug carriers. The membrane viscoelasticity described by appropriate constitutive model is related to kinetic of drug release in order to whole process optimization. Furthermore, chapter will bring review of developed hybrid drug delivery vehicles of erythrocyte membranes as natural bio-derivative material, and nanoparticles, mainly made of synthetic material, whose combined advantages serve as immunologically non-invasive drug delivery platform. The advantages and drawbacks are specifically summarized to get critical point of view on existing and future medical applications of erythrocyte membrane as drug carriers. As an example of complexity in research toward development of such erythrocyte membrane based drug delivery systems starting from animal erythrocyte, morphological, biochemical and drug release profile assessment will be reviewed.

Chapter 4 - The electrochemical properties of blood cells play an important role in maintaining cell stability and biological function, and they are the deciding factor in the interaction of blood cells with both foreign materials and bodily tissues. Therefore, it is very important to investigate the electrochemical behavior of blood cells. The application of an electrochemical approach to rationalizing blood cell behavior in contact with foreign electrical conductors opens up opportunities for the development of novel analytical and diagnostic methods. The present work investigated the electrochemical behavior of erythrocytes (red blood cells) at platinum, carbonaceous, and optically transparent electrodes via polarization and coulometric measurements. Electrochemical activity of red blood cells was shown in both cathodic and anodic potential ranges of the above electrodes. The interaction of blood cells with the charged electrode surface was accompanied by electron transfer and changes in the morphology of cell membranes. The directionality of electron transfer and concomitant cell morphology changes were found to be dependent on the electrode potential. The order of magnitude of the quantity of electrons transferred between erythrocytes and electrodes was determined, and potential ranges showing indifference of the electrode toward red blood cells were identified. These results can be used to develop a method for evaluating the condition of normal and pathological erythrocytes, as well as to test novel materials for hemocompatibility.

Chapter 1

RESEARCH ADVANCES IN ERYTHROID DEVELOPMENT FROM HUMAN PLURIPOTENT STEM CELLS

Yijin Chen[1], Bin Mao[1], PhD, Jia Feng[1], Yonggang Zhang[1], PhD and Feng Ma[1,2,], PhD*

[1]Institute of Blood Transfusion, Chinese Academy of Medical Sciences & Peking Union Medical College (CAMS & PUMC), Chengdu, China
[2]State Key Lab of Experimental Hematology, Institute of Hematology and Blood Diseases Hospital, CAMS & PUMC, Tianjin, China

ABSTRACT

Erythroid cells play an essential role in whole life of mammals, particularly in supporting the growth and survival of the embryo/fetus. Human erythropoiesis has already been precisely described in adult but not yet in embryo. Human pluripotent stem cells (hPSCs) are of great potential for tissue substitutes (for example, blood cells) and to cure various congenital disorders. So far, many laboratories have reported that mature erythrocytes could be efficiently generated from hPSCs using

---

* Corresponding Author's E-mail: mafeng@hotmail.co.jp.

different methods. Recent reports show that hPSC-derived hematopoiesis follows two different pathways, and erythrocytes as the earliest developed blood cells have a unique developmental pathway through hematopoiesis. In this chapter, we summarize advances in hPSC-derived erythroid development and molecular regulatory mechanism. These researches may provide a new perspective on human embryo erythropoiesis and a possible treatment for some hematological diseases. The critical problems need to be solved and the research prospects of this field will also be addressed at the end of the chapter.

Keywords: hPSCs, HSC-independent, erythropoiesis

INTRODUCTION

Red blood cells (RBCs) are one of the most important cell types that fulfil basic biological functions in human as well as in other species. They play a crucial role in whole life, particularly in carrying oxygen and supporting the growth and survival of the embryo/fetus. Besides, it is reported that parts of erythrocytes with special marker have unique immunologic function in both mouse and human [1, 2]. Erythrocytes are derived from hematopoietic stem/progenitor cells [3, 4], while they originated from two developmental waves; one from early yolk sacs that forming the earliest blood cells including large nucleated erythroblasts, macrophages, megakaryocytes, mast cells and some granulocytes; and the other from adult-type hematopoietic stem cells (HSCs) in bone marrow. The development of human adult-type erythrocytes has already been precisely described, but not yet in embryo because of the ethical and law restrictions that hamper the research on human embryos. Human pluripotent stem cells (hPSCs) are of great potential for regenerative medicine (for example, blood cells) and to cure various congenital disorders. hPSC-derived erythrocytes also offer an ideal model to study human embryonic erythropoiesis *in vitro*. So far, many laboratories have reported that mature erythrocytes could be efficiently generated from hPSCs through the formation of embryo bodies (EBs), or co-cultures with stromal cells. Recent reports show that hPSC-derived hematopoiesis follows two different pathways namely HSC-dependent and –independent pathways. Erythrocytes as the earliest developed blood cells have a unique developmental pattern through both HSC-independent and –dependent hematopoiesis. Evidences show that hPSC-derived early wave of erythroid development is largely different from that of HSC-derived ones. Thus, the question of whether those HSC- independent erythrocytes have endowed with definitive function even extend in adult stage is a critical issue to be elucidated. Some works have focused on the molecular regulation of hPSC-derived erythroid development. Molecular biology analysis such as RNA sequencing suggests different transcriptome in HSC-independent and dependent erythropoiesis. Since hPSC-derived erythrocytes have great prospects in translational medicine, to clarify their methodology and molecular regulatory mechanism is very important.

In this chapter, we summarize advances in hPSC-derived erythroid development and its molecular regulatory mechanism. These researches may provide both new perspectives on human embryo erythropoiesis and possible cures for hematological diseases. The vital problems need to be solved and the research prospects of this field will also be addressed at the end of the chapter.

METHODS OF GAINING HPSC-DERIVED ERYTHROCYTES

Most studies obtain human erythrocytes *in vitro* by directly culturing hematopoietic stem and progenitor cells (HSPCs) derived from cord blood (CB), bone marrow (BM) or peripheral blood (PB) [5-9]. However, these resources are limited and erythrocytes generated from them are also immunogenic. hPSCs have abilities of self-renewal and derivation of all kind of cells, so the method of generating hPSC-derived erythroid cells attracts more and more attentions. In the last decades, a lot of works have established methods to gain large number of erythroid from hPSCs.

As early as 2001, erythroid progenitor cells were successfully obtained from hESCs by co-culturing with S17, the mouse bone marrow stromal cell line, and C166, a yolk-sac endothelial cell line, and both two different stromal cell co-cultured-derived erythroid cells were glycophorin A+ (GPA+) and expressed adult β-globin [10]. Studies on erythroid cells derived from hPSCs have provided important information about human erythropoiesis in embryo.

During the embryo development, fetal liver (FL) plays an essential role in hematopoiesis, especially in erythropoiesis. The progenitor cells with definitive erythroid potential are found in the fetal liver in mouse embryo [11]. Similar to this finding in mouse, these progenitor cells are also detected in the fetal liver of the human embryo [12]. Therefore, fetal liver stromal cells (FLSCs) might facilitate the method of erythroid cells production *in vitro* [13, 14]. In 2005, Caihong Qiu et al. [15] reported a more efficient method to induce differentiation from hESCs into erythroid progenitor cells by co-culturing with FH-B-hTERT cells, the human fetal liver stromal cell line. Moreover, in 2008, Ma F, et al. [16] gained enormous erythroblasts from hESCs through co-culturing with mFLSCs, and these cells with adult β-globin expression had normally oxygen carrying capacity, sufficient glucose-6-phosphate dehydrogenase activity and could enucleate effectively. Then in 2010, Yu-xiao Liu et al. [17] succeeded in differentiating human embryoid body (hEB) generated of human hESCs to functional mature erythroid cells with both embryonic and adult globin expression, by treating with cell extract from human fetal liver tissue and co-culturing with hFLSCs. This research provided a humanized way to get functional erythroid cells from hESCs. Then, they facilitated this method by establishing hFLSCs which was expressing erythropoietin (EPO) [18].

In addition, the mouse bone marrow stromal cell line OP-9 is another important stromal cell line to help gaining erythroid cells from hESCs. However, it is reported that in the OP9 co-cultured system, adult globin expression in hESCs/hiPSC-derived erythroid cells was lower when compared with embryonic and fetal globin [19, 20]. Recent study has found that not only OP9 co-culture, but factors secreted by OP9 cells in isolation increase the proliferative potential of PB-derived adult erythroid cells by delaying differentiation [21]. Besides, stromal-free culture system is another strategy to generate erythrocytes from hPSCs [22-24]. Under stromal and serum-free culture conditions, Lu S. J. et al. [25] successfully obtained large quantity production of enucleated erythroid cells, although these cells have oxygen-carrying capacities, they still mainly express embryonic globin.

Table 1. Methods of generating erythrocytes from hPSCs

Starting cell type	Approach	Hemoglobin expression	References
ES cells	S17 or C166 co-culture	α, β, δ	[10]
ES cells	EB co-culture on mFLSCs	β, ε, γ	[13]
ES cells	mFLSCs co-culture	ε, γ	[14]
ES cells	FH-B-hTERT or S17 co-culture	ε, γ	[15]
ES cells	mFLSCs co-culture	β, ε, γ	[16]
ES cells	hFLSCs co-culture	α, β, ζ, ε, γ	[17, 18]
iPS cells	OP9 or MS-5 co-culture	ε, γ	[19]
ES cells	OP9 or MS-5 co-culture	α, ζ, γ	[20]
ES cells	EB	β, ε, γ	[22]
ES cells	EB	ζ, ε, γ	[23]
ES and iPS cells	EB	α, ε, ζ, γ	[24]
ES cells	EB	β, ζ, ε, γ	[25]
iPS cells derived patients with sickle cell disease	OP9 co-culture	β, ε, γ	[29]
hPSC	immortalized cell line (c-MYC and BCL-XL)	ε, γ	[30]
iPS cells	immortalized cell line (TAL-1)	α, β, γ	[31]

Human induce pluripotent stem cells (iPSCs) derived from adult somatic cells is another resource for scalable production of erythrocytes *in vitro*. iPSCs are more efficiently differentiated to mature erythrocytes due to epigenetic memory [26]. Besides, iPSCs derived from patients with hematologic disease provide an effective model to study patient-tailored hematopoietic disorders. However, iPSCs-derived erythroid cells predominantly produce embryonic globin with little adult globin expression [19, 27, 28]. Recently, some researchers have succeeded in generating erythroid cells with β-globin expression from iPSCs derived from sickle cell disease patients [29].

Some recent studies focus on establishing immortalized erythroid progenitor cell lines. In 2013, Hirose S et al. [30] transduced c-MYC and BCL-XL into hPSC-derived multipotent hematopoietic progenitor cells, named imERYPCs, to obtain immortalized erythroblasts. However, these erythroblasts mainly display fetal-type globin and have a very low enucleation ratio. Kurita et al. established immortalized cell lines by using UCB-derived HSPCs and hiPSCs [31]. These cell lines produce functional globin and express erythroid-specific markers, but the efficiency of enucleated erythroid cells production still remains to be improved [31].

Methods related to hPSC-derived erythrocytes are listed in Table 1.

THE DEVELOPMENT OF HUMAN ERYTHROCYTES

hPSCs make it possible to uncover various normal or diseased mechanisms in early human development. To mimic hematopoiesis in human embryo, various *in vitro* differentiation systems have been used, such as EB forming [23, 32] or co-culture with hematopoietic niche-derived stromal cell lines, like OP9 [19], AGM-S3 [33, 34] and m/hFLSCs [16, 17, 35]. Based on these culture systems, researchers try to clarify the details of early development of human erythroid cells using hESCs as a model.

Hematopoiesis in Mouse or Human Embryo

In mouse model, there are three waves of hematopoiesis during embryo development. The first wave called primitive hematopoiesis that originates at embryonic day E7.0 at Yolk Sac (YS), producing large erythroblasts with embryonic globin expression [36]. Subsequently, the second wave, termed pro-definitive wave, occurs in different sites of the mouse embryo (YS, embryo proper and allantois) [37]. This wave generates erythroid/myeloid progenitors (EMPs) and EMP-derived definitive erythroblasts expressing adult globin [38, 39]. These two different ways of hematopoiesis also named HSC-independent hematopoiesis [37]. Recent work indicates that some tissue-resident blood cells, such as B-1a cells [40], macrophage [41], derived from this process have an important function in adult, suggesting that HSC-independent hematopoiesis plays an essential role in embryo development. The third wave, named HSC-dependent hematopoiesis, produces transplantable HSCs that can give rise to all mature blood cell at E10.5 in the AGM region [42].

Similar to mouse, three waves of hematopoiesis are detected during human embryo development. In the 20th century, some studies on human embryo showed that primitive erythroblasts first arose at 18-20 days of gestation, and these cells with embryonic globin expression were the only circulating erythroid cells from 3 to 6 weeks of gestation [43]. These primitive erythroid cells undergo terminal maturation in placenta under assist from macrophages [44]. Interestingly, the erythroid burst-forming units (BFU-E) were first detected in the YS as early as 4-5 weeks gestation [12]. Then, they have a dramatic depletion, while they can easily detected in the bloodstream and their number have a striking increase in the FL as soon as it began to form as an organ [12]. These data suggest that the early BFU-Es are generated in YS, then migrating to FL. Subsequently, hematopoietic progenitors were first found at 27 days of gestation as small groups of 2-3 cells then rapidly form clusters of thousand of cells [45, 46]. These data support the conclusion that definitive erythropoiesis has two developmental origins [43]. However, it's difficult to study human embryo erythropoiesis systematically due to the ethical restrictions. So, hPSCs provide a perfect tool to fulfil the map of human erythropoiesis in embryo.

Research on Erythroid Development Using hESCs

Coincided with what has been found in human embryo research, three waves of hematopoiesis are also detected during the culture of hESCs in hematopoietic differentiation condition.

Studies of hESCs-derived human primitive erythroblast have showed that they express embryonic globin and CD31$^+$ with GPA$^+$, while definitive erythroblasts express CD36$^+$ with GPA+ [47]. Moreover, these erythroblasts need undergo a maturation switch: hemoglobin Gower I ($\zeta_2\varepsilon_2$) to hemoglobin Gower II ($\alpha_2\varepsilon_2$) [48] similar to that happened in embryos. Besides, EPO is absolutely required for them, and an inverse correlation between FLI1 and both KLF1 and EPOR is detected during primitive erythroid differentiation, similar to definitive hematopoiesis [20, 49]. Some recent works shows that the cytoskeleton of primitive and definitive erythroid lineages share common structural features [43, 50]. Transcriptional regulation in primitive erythroid cells was widely reported in mouse. Some transcriptional factors, like GATA1, EKLF, Erf, play key roles as same as that in definitive erythroid cells [4, 51-53]. However, the similar result has not been reported in hPSC-derived primitive and definitive erythroblasts. Recently, researchers found that hiPSCs-derived primitive erythroblasts fail to express hallmark red cell transcripts of adult erythropoiesis [47].

The HSC-independent definitive erythroid derived from hESCs could also be observed during the hematopoietic differentiation. In our laboratory previous work, we found that numerous erythroblasts with β-globin expression were developed before the emergence of HSPCs, and these cells have a different developmental way from CB-derived erythroid cells (Figure 1) [34]. However, little has been known about this wave of definitive erythroid derived from hESCs.

Although erythroid cells can be obtained from hPSCs [10, 15-17, 21, 25, 29-31], a detailed molecular roadmap of developmental erythropoiesis has not been previously described from hPSCs. It is difficult to sort primitive and definitive erythroblasts from hPSCs during culturing by the expression of β-globin. In 2014, Christopher M. Sturgeon, et al. established selective differentiation strategies for the generation of primitive or definitive hematopoietic progenitors from hPSCs by Wnt-β-catenin manipulation [54]. A recent work distinguishes primitive from definitive erythroblasts by expressing $CD31^+GPA^+$ and $CD36^+GPA^+$ respectively [47]. This work also shows that there is a high relationship at a molecular and functional level between hiPSCs-derived erythroblasts generating from hematopoietic progenitors and CB $CD34^+$-derived erythroblasts [47].

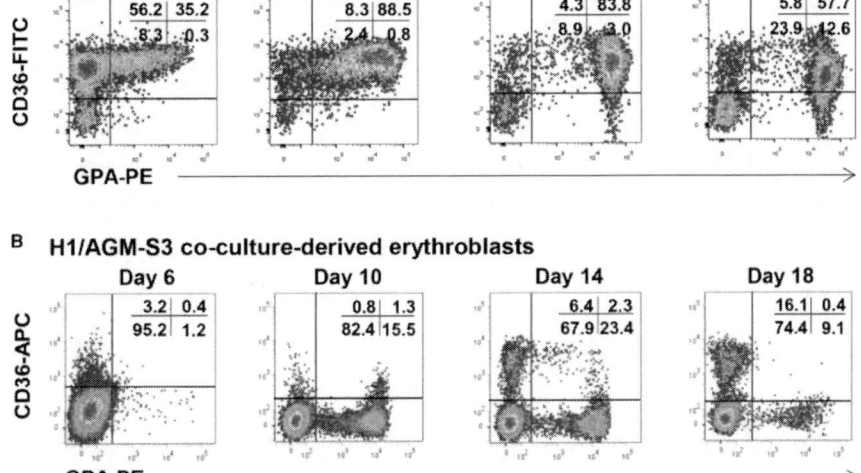

Representative flow cytometry profiles showing expression of CD36 on GPA^+ cells derived from A) hCB-$CD34^+$ HSPCs and B) H1/AGM-S3 co-culture.
Adapted from Mao Bin, et al. Stem Cell Reports, 2016.

Figure 1. Expression process of CD36 on erythroid cells of different origins [34].

Taken together, these studies indicate that hPSCs have ability of simulating various stages of development erythropoiesis. Primitive and definitive erythropoiesis can both be detected from differentiation of hPSCs, and these processes are similar to those in mouse/human embryos.

MOLECULAR REGULATION OF hPSC-DERIVED ERYTHROID DEVELOPMENT

Despite the difficulty to distinguish different stages of development erythropoiesis, the molecular regulation was studied in hPSC-derived erythroblasts.

The roles of several cytokines are crucial in erythropoiesis. One of the most well researched cytokines is EPO. EPO is widely needed in erythropoiesis. Researches based on mouse and hCB CD34$^+$ cells found that erythroid cells require EPO for survival, especially for generating colony-forming unit erythroid (CFU-E) and burst-forming unit erythroid (BFU-E) cells [9, 49]. Similarly, EPO is absolutely required for hESCs-derived primitive human embryonic erythropoiesis, and there is synergism between EPO and IL-3 [20, 49, 55]. Another well-researched cytokine for erythroid development is stem cell factor (SCF) which the ligand for c-kit that binds to c-kit receptor. SCF has a synergy with EPO in mouse and hCB CD-34$^+$ cells-derived erythropoiesis [9, 56, 57], but in contrast to that in hPSC-derived ones. There was a reduced expression of c-kit during erythroid differentiation from hPSCs [20, 58]. Besides, VEGF-A$_{165}$ has an important function in erythropoiesis. A study found that the presence of this cytokine enhanced the *in vitro* self-renewal potential of erythroid progenitor cells [22].

Transcriptional factors play an essential role in erythroid development, and the commitment of erythroid lineage and subsequent maturation is ultimately controlled by them that tightly regulate erythroid-specific gene expression networks [57]. The genome-wide transcription dynamics and large-scale transcriptional analysis show that the predominantly up-regulated genes upon differentiation are erythroid/hematopoietic genes, such as GATA1/2, KLF1, and TAL1/SCL [59-61]. Those genes are crucial in erythropoiesis both in mouse and human adults [57, 62-67] and they show similar functions in hPSC-derived erythropoiesis [20, 22, 61, 68]. These data indicate a stable pattern of gene expression during erythropoiesis. However, the expression of some transcriptional factors related with enucleation, like BCL11A, are different between hPSC-derived and adults erythroid cells [58]. But this difference in expression of BCL11A is quite consistent with the specification of primitive erythroid cells [58], suggesting that hPSC-derived erythroblasts still remain primitive property.

The function of non-coding RNAs, including microRNA and long non-coding RNA (lncRNA), is increasingly noticed in erythropoiesis. miR-30a, which increasingly expressed during erythroid differentiation both in mouse and human [69, 70], can increase the percent of enucleated erythroid cells in hESCs cultures [71]. Other microRNAs have also been reported to have functions in erythropoiesis. For example, miR-142-3p, miR142-5p, miR-146a and miR-451 are dynamically changed during erythropoiesis of hESCs [72]. miRs-126/126* has an inhibitory role in erythropoiesis from hESCs [73]. LncRNA also plays a pivotal role in erythropoiesis. Some erythroid specific lncRNAs can promote erythroid cells maturation and inhibits apoptosis of mature erythrocytes in both mouse and human [57, 74-76]. However, there are few researches on lncRNAs in erythropoiesis from hPSCs.

CONCLUSION

In past decades, it's a general thinking that there are three waves of hematopoiesis (primitive, first definitive and definitive hematopoiesis) in embryo. However, recent works suggest that it's not a single, fixed hierarchical order during hematopoietic development [37, 77]. Under this finding, it comes up with a new aspect on hematopoiesis — HSC-independent and –dependent hematopoiesis (Figure 2) [37]. The former can generate either short-lived (primitive erythroid cells) or long-lived (tissue-resident macrophages) cells, and the the latter can produce all the adult blood cells [37]. Notably, long-lived HSC-independent blood cells have ability to reside in tissues. For example, HSC-independent macrophages become microglia in the brain, and these cells are different from HSC-derived in function and gene expression [41, 78]. Besides, HSC-independent hematopoiesis also can generate some specialized blood cells, like B-1a cells [40] and HSC- independent T cells [79, 80]. Interestingly, a work shows that there are unique tumor-inducible erythroblast-like cells both in mouse and human with hepatocellular carcinoma (HCC), and these cells have a tumor-promoting ability [81]. Interestingly, this study found that these cells may be derived from megakaryocyte-erythroid progenitor cells (MEP) [81]. This study suggests that the existence of tissue-resident erythroblasts and these cells may have a unique function in adults. HSC-independent blood cells may play an unsubstitutable role in development of embryo, and provide potential approaches to obtain the functional blood cells *in vitro*.

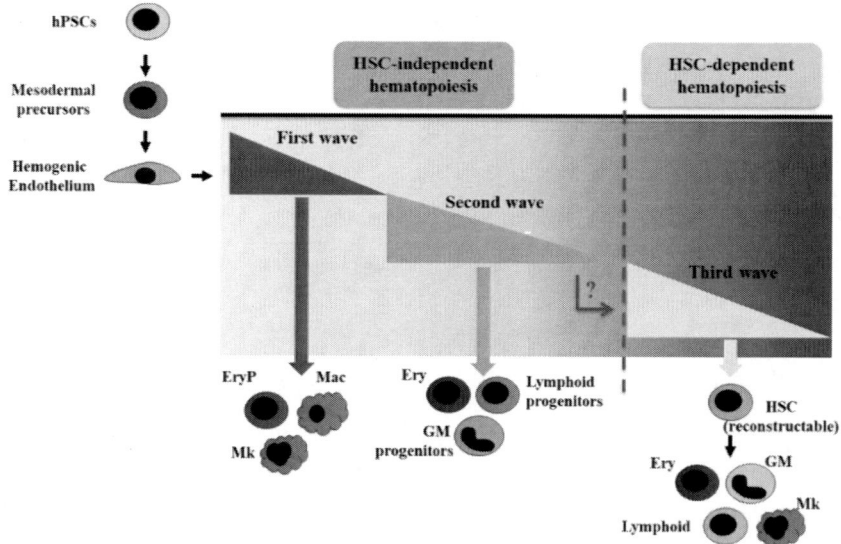

Figure 2. HSC-independent and HSC-dependent hematopoietic lineages from hPSCs.

HSC-independent hematopoietic lineages generated in the first wave and second wave during hPSCs differentiation. These cells are either primitive such as primitive erythroid cells, or definitive with specialized function, such as tissue-resident macrophages. HSC-dependent hematopoiesis can give rise to the most of blood cells found in the tissues and circulation of adults. HE, Hemogenic endothelial cells; EryP, primitive erythrocytes; Mac, macrophage; Mk, megakaryocyte; Ery, erythrocytes; GM, granulocyte-macrophage hPSCs have provided potential tools of studying early developmental events of human embryonic hematopoiesis. As a result of extensive studies, it's still difficult to observe a complete HSC-independent hematopoiesis from hPSCs. Therefore, a suitable hematopoietic environment may have an essential impact on hPSCs differentiation. Sequentially co-culturing with stromal cells derived from embryonic hematopoietic niche, such as YS, AGM and FL, may help observe a similar process in erythropoiesis from hPSCs to that in embryo. Moreover, cytoskeletal network and molecular regulation in hPSC-derived HSC-independent and –dependent erythropoiesis are also critical to understand. The study of HSC-independent erythrocytes will probably undergo substantial refinement in the coming years.

REFERENCES

[1] Elahi, S; et al. (2013). Immunosuppressive CD71+ erythroid cells compromise neonatal host defence against infection. *Nature*, 504(7478), p. 158-62.
[2] Namdar, A; et al. (2017). CD71(+) erythroid suppressor cells impair adaptive immunity against Bordetella pertussis. *Sci Rep*, 7(1), p. 7728.
[3] Palis, J. (2008). Ontogeny of erythropoiesis. *Curr Opin Hematol*, 15(3), p. 155-61.
[4] Baron, MH; Vacaru, A; Nieves, J. (2013). Erythroid development in the mammalian embryo. *Blood Cells Mol Dis*, 51(4), p. 213-9.
[5] Malik, P; et al. (1998). An *in vitro* model of human red blood cell production from hematopoietic progenitor cells. *Blood*, 91(8), p. 2664-71.
[6] Panzenbock, B; et al. (1998). Growth and differentiation of human stem cell factor/erythropoietin-dependent erythroid progenitor cells *in vitro*. *Blood*, 92(10), p. 3658-68.

[7] Migliaccio, G; et al. (2002). *In vitro* mass production of human erythroid cells from the blood of normal donors and of thalassemic patients. *Blood Cells Mol Dis*, 28(2), p. 169-80.

[8] Neildez-Nguyen, TM; et al. (2002). Human erythroid cells produced ex vivo at large scale differentiate into red blood cells *in vivo*. *Nat Biotechnol*, 20(5), p. 467-72.

[9] Li, J; et al. (2014). Isolation and transcriptome analyses of human erythroid progenitors: BFU-E and CFU-E. *Blood*, 124(24), p. 3636-45.

[10] Kaufman, DS; et al. (2001). Hematopoietic colony-forming cells derived from human embryonic stem cells. *Proc Natl Acad Sci U S A*, 98(19), p. 10716-21.

[11] Lux, CT; et al. (2008). All primitive and definitive hematopoietic progenitor cells emerging before E10 in the mouse embryo are products of the yolk sac. *Blood*, 111(7), p. 3435-8.

[12] Migliaccio, G; et al. (1986). Human embryonic hemopoiesis. Kinetics of progenitors and precursors underlying the yolk sac—liver transition. *J Clin Invest*, 78(1), p. 51-60.

[13] Lee, KY; et al. (2011). Fetal stromal niches enhance human embryonic stem cell-derived hematopoietic differentiation and globin switch. *Stem Cells Dev*, 20(1), p. 31-8.

[14] Ledran, MH; et al. (2008) Efficient hematopoietic differentiation of human embryonic stem cells on stromal cells derived from hematopoietic niches. *Cell Stem Cell*, 3(1), p. 85-98.

[15] Qiu, C; et al. (2005). Differentiation of human embryonic stem cells into hematopoietic cells by coculture with human fetal liver cells recapitulates the globin switch that occurs early in development. *Exp Hematol*, 33(12), p. 1450-8.

[16] Ma, F; et al. (2008). Generation of functional erythrocytes from human embryonic stem cell-derived definitive hematopoiesis. *Proc Natl Acad Sci U S A*, 105(35), p. 13087-92.

[17] Liu, YX; et al. (2010). Production of erythriod cells from human embryonic stem cells by fetal liver cell extract treatment. *BMC Dev Biol*, 10, p. 85.

[18] Yang, C; et al. (2012). Human fetal liver stromal cells expressing erythropoietin promote hematopoietic development from human embryonic stem cells. *Cell Reprogram*, 14(1), p. 88-97.

[19] Dias, J; et al. (2011). Generation of red blood cells from human induced pluripotent stem cells. *Stem Cells Dev*, 20(9), p. 1639-47.

[20] Klimchenko, O; et al. (2009). A common bipotent progenitor generates the erythroid and megakaryocyte lineages in embryonic stem cell-derived primitive hematopoiesis. *Blood*, 114(8), p. 1506-17.

[21] Trakarnsanga, K; et al. (2018). Secretory factors from OP9 stromal cells delay differentiation and increase the expansion potential of adult erythroid cells *in vitro*. *Sci Rep*, 8(1), p. 1983.

[22] Cerdan, C; Rouleau, A; Bhatia, M. (2004). VEGF-A165 augments erythropoietic development from human embryonic stem cells. *Blood*, 103(7), p. 2504-12.

[23] Chang, KH; et al. (2006). Definitive-like erythroid cells derived from human embryonic stem cells coexpress high levels of embryonic and fetal globins with little or no adult globin. *Blood*, 108(5), p. 1515-23.

[24] Lapillonne, H; et al. (2010). Red blood cell generation from human induced pluripotent stem cells: perspectives for transfusion medicine. *Haematologica*, 2010, 95(10), p. 1651-9.

[25] Lu, SJ; et al. (2008). Biologic properties and enucleation of red blood cells from human embryonic stem cells. *Blood*, 112(12), p. 4475-84.

[26] Kim, K; et al. (2010). Epigenetic memory in induced pluripotent stem cells. *Nature*, 467(7313), p. 285-90.

[27] Vo, LT; Daley, GQ. (2015). De novo generation of HSCs from somatic and pluripotent stem cell sources. *Blood* 125(17), p. 2641-8.

[28] Chou, BK; et al. (2011). Efficient human iPS cell derivation by a non-integrating plasmid from blood cells with unique epigenetic and gene expression signatures. *Cell Res*, 21(3), p. 518-29.

[29] Uchida, N; et al. (2017). Efficient Generation of beta-Globin-Expressing Erythroid Cells Using Stromal Cell-Derived Induced Pluripotent Stem Cells from Patients with Sickle Cell Disease. *Stem Cells*, 35(3), p. 586-596.

[30] Hirose, S; et al. (2013). Immortalization of erythroblasts by c-MYC and BCL-XL enables large-scale erythrocyte production from human pluripotent stem cells. *Stem Cell Reports*, 1(6), p. 499-508.

[31] Kurita, R; et al. (2013). Establishment of immortalized human erythroid progenitor cell lines able to produce enucleated red blood cells. *PLoS One*, 8(3), p. e59890.

[32] Chang, KH; et al. (2010). Globin phenotype of erythroid cells derived from human induced pluripotent stem cells. *Blood*, 115(12), p. 2553-4.

[33] Sakashita, K; et al. (2015). *In vitro* expansion of CD34(+)CD38(-) cells under stimulation with hematopoietic growth factors on AGM-S3 cells in juvenile myelomonocytic leukemia. *Leukemia*, 29(3), p. 606-14.

[34] Mao, B; et al. (2016). Early Development of Definitive Erythroblasts from Human Pluripotent Stem Cells Defined by Expression of Glycophorin A/CD235a, CD34, and CD36. *Stem Cell Reports*, 7(5), p. 869-883.

[35] Ma, F; et al. (2007). Novel method for efficient production of multipotential hematopoietic progenitors from human embryonic stem cells. *Int J Hematol*, 85(5), p. 371-9.

[36] Ferkowicz, MJ; et al. (2003). CD41 expression defines the onset of primitive and definitive hematopoiesis in the murine embryo. *Development*, 130(18), p. 4393-403.

[37] Dzierzak, E; Bigas, A. (2018). Blood Development: Hematopoietic Stem Cell Dependence and Independence. *Cell Stem Cell*, 22(5), p. 639-651.

[38] Frame, JM; McGrath, KE; Palis, J. (2013). Erythro-myeloid progenitors: "definitive" hematopoiesis in the conceptus prior to the emergence of hematopoietic stem cells. *Blood Cells Mol Dis*, 51(4), p. 220-5.

[39] McGrath, KE; et al. (2015). Distinct Sources of Hematopoietic Progenitors Emerge before HSCs and Provide Functional Blood Cells in the Mammalian Embryo. *Cell Rep*, 11(12), p. 1892-904.

[40] Hadland, BK; et al. (2017). A Common Origin for B-1a and B-2 Lymphocytes in Clonal Pre- Hematopoietic Stem Cells. *Stem Cell Reports*, 8(6), p. 1563-1572.

[41] Ginhoux, F; et al. (2010). Fate mapping analysis reveals that adult microglia derive from primitive macrophages. *Science*, 330(6005), p. 841-5.

[42] de Bruijn, MF; et al. (2000) Definitive hematopoietic stem cells first develop within the major arterial regions of the mouse embryo. *EMBO J*, 19(11), p. 2465-74.

[43] Palis, J. (2014). Primitive and definitive erythropoiesis in mammals. *Front Physiol*, 5, p. 3.

[44] Van Handel, B; et al. (2010) The first trimester human placenta is a site for terminal maturation of primitive erythroid cells. *Blood*, 116(17), p. 3321-30.

[45] Tavian, M; et al. (1996). Aorta-associated CD34+ hematopoietic cells in the early human embryo. *Blood*, 87(1), p. 67-72.

[46] Julien, E; El Omar, R; Tavian, M. (2016). Origin of the hematopoietic system in the human embryo. *FEBS Lett*, 590(22), p. 3987-4001.

[47] Razaq, MA; et al. (2017). A molecular roadmap of definitive erythropoiesis from human induced pluripotent stem cells. *Br J Haematol*, 176(6), p. 971-983.

[48] Qiu, C; et al. (2008). Globin switches in yolk sac-like primitive and fetal-like definitive red blood cells produced from human embryonic stem cells. *Blood*, 111(4), p. 2400-8.

[49] Malik, J; et al. (2013). Erythropoietin critically regulates the terminal maturation of murine and human primitive erythroblasts. *Haematologica*, 98(11), p. 1778-87.

[50] Ponnusamy, S; et al. (2012). Membrane proteins of human fetal primitive nucleated red blood cells. *J Proteomics*, 75(18), p. 5762-73.

[51] Fujiwara, Y; et al. (2004). Functional overlap of GATA-1 and GATA-2 in primitive hematopoietic development. *Blood*, 103(2), p. 583-5.

[52] Hodge, D; et al. (2006). A global role for EKLF in definitive and primitive erythropoiesis. *Blood*, 107(8), p. 3359-70.

[53] Peraki, I; Palis, J; Mavrothalassitis, G. (2017). The Ets2 Repressor Factor (Erf) Is Required for Effective Primitive and Definitive Hematopoiesis. *Mol Cell Biol*, 37(19).

[54] Sturgeon, CM; et al. (2014). Wnt signaling controls the specification of definitive and primitive hematopoiesis from human pluripotent stem cells. *Nat Biotechnol*, 32(6), p. 554-61.

[55] Lin, CS; et al. (1996). Differential effects of an erythropoietin receptor gene disruption on primitive and definitive erythropoiesis. *Genes Dev*, 10(2), p. 154-64.

[56] Wu, H; et al. (1995). Interaction of the erythropoietin and stem-cell-factor receptors. *Nature*, 377(6546), p. 242-6.

[57] Nandakumar, SK; Ulirsch, JC; Sankaran, VG. (2016). Advances in understanding erythropoiesis: evolving perspectives. *Br J Haematol*, 173(2), p. 206-18.

[58] Merryweather-Clarke, AT; et al. (2016). Distinct gene expression program dynamics during erythropoiesis from human induced pluripotent stem cells compared with adult and cord blood progenitors. *BMC Genomics*, 17(1), p. 817.

[59] Yang, Y; et al. (2013). Transcriptome dynamics during human erythroid differentiation and development. *Genomics*, 102(5-6), p. 431-441.

[60] Lu, SJ; et al. (2007). GeneChip analysis of human embryonic stem cell differentiation into hemangioblasts: an in silico dissection of mixed phenotypes. *Genome Biol*, 8(11), p. R240.

[61] Yung, S; et al. (2011). Large-scale transcriptional profiling and functional assays reveal important roles for Rho-GTPase signalling and SCL during haematopoietic differentiation of human embryonic stem cells. *Hum Mol Genet*, 20(24), p. 4932-46.

[62] Moriguchi, T; Yamamoto, M. (2014). A regulatory network governing Gata1 and Gata2 gene transcription orchestrates erythroid lineage differentiation. *Int J Hematol*, 100(5), p. 417-24.

[63] Ohneda, K; Yamamoto, M. (2002). Roles of hematopoietic transcription factors GATA-1 and GATA-2 in the development of red blood cell lineage. *Acta Haematol*, 108(4), p. 237-45.

[64] Barminko, J; Reinholt, B; Baron, MH. (2016). Development and differentiation of the erythroid lineage in mammals. *Dev Comp Immunol*, 58, p. 18-29.

[65] Katsumura, KR; Bresnick, EH; Group, GFM. (2017). The GATA factor revolution in hematology. *Blood*, 129(15), p. 2092-2102.

[66] Sankaran, VG; et al. (2012). Exome sequencing identifies GATA1 mutations resulting in Diamond-Blackfan anemia. *J Clin Invest*, 122(7), p. 2439-43.

[67] Xu, J; et al. (2012). Combinatorial assembly of developmental stage-specific enhancers controls gene expression programs during human erythropoiesis. *Dev Cell*, 23(4), p. 796-811.

[68] Yang, CT; et al. (2017). Activation of KLF1 Enhances the Differentiation and Maturation of Red Blood Cells from Human Pluripotent Stem Cells. *Stem Cells*, 35(4), p. 886-897.

[69] Choong, ML; Yang, HH; McNiece, I. (2007). MicroRNA expression profiling during human cord blood-derived CD34 cell erythropoiesis. *Exp Hematol*, 35(4), p. 551-64.

[70] Zhan, M; et al. (2007). MicroRNA expression dynamics during murine and human erythroid differentiation. *Exp Hematol*, 35(7), p. 1015-25.

[71] Rouzbeh, S; et al. (2015). Molecular signature of erythroblast enucleation in human embryonic stem cells. *Stem Cells*, 33(8), p. 2431-41.

[72] Jin, HL; et al. (2012). Dynamic expression of specific miRNAs during erythroid differentiation of human embryonic stem cells. *Mol Cells*, 34(2), p. 177-83.

[73] Huang, X; et al. (2011). Regulated expression of microRNAs-126/126* inhibits erythropoiesis from human embryonic stem cells. *Blood*, 117(7), p. 2157-65.

[74] Li, W; et al. (2018). Long non-coding RNAs in hematopoietic regulation. *Cell Regen* (Lond), 7(2), p. 27-32.

[75] Hu, W; et al. (2011). Long noncoding RNA-mediated anti-apoptotic activity in murine erythroid terminal differentiation. *Genes Dev*, 25(24), p. 2573-8.

[76] Alvarez-Dominguez, JR; et al. (2014). Global discovery of erythroid long noncoding RNAs reveals novel regulators of red cell maturation. *Blood*, 123(4), p. 570-81.

[77] McGrath, KE; Frame, JM; Palis, J. (2015). Early hematopoiesis and macrophage development. *Semin Immunol*, 27(6), p. 379-87.

[78] Perdiguero, EG; et al. (2015). The Origin of Tissue-Resident Macrophages: When an Erythro-myeloid Progenitor Is an Erythro-myeloid Progenitor. *Immunity*, 43(6), p. 1023-4.

[79] Yoshimoto, M; et al. (2012). Autonomous murine T-cell progenitor production in the extra-embryonic yolk sac before HSC emergence. *Blood*, 119(24), p. 5706-14.

[80] Luis, TC; et al. (2016). Initial seeding of the embryonic thymus by immune-restricted lympho-myeloid progenitors. *Nat Immunol*, 17(12), p. 1424-1435.

[81] Han, Y; et al. (2018). Tumor-Induced Generation of Splenic Erythroblast-like Ter-Cells Promotes Tumor Progression. *Cell*, 173(3), p. 634-648 e12.

In: Erythrocytes
Editor: Katy Jorissen

ISBN: 978-1-53615-914-1
© 2019 Nova Science Publishers, Inc.

Chapter 2

ERYTHROCYTE DISORDERS: CAUSES AND CLINICAL OUTCOMES

R. Vani, PhD and R. Soumya, PhD

Department of Biotechnology,
JAIN (Deemed-to-be University), Bengaluru,
Karnataka, India

ABSTRACT

Erythrocytes or red blood cells (RBCs) are important constituents of blood, whose main function is to transport oxygen to tissues through hemoglobin. These cells are produced by erythropoiesis, mature in 8 days and have a life span of 120 days. Erythrocytes are enucleate, possess a specialized cell membrane and depend on glycolysis and pentose phosphate pathways for energy.

Erythrocytes are well equipped to carry out their functions due to a dynamic cell membrane, their inherent shape & lack of organelles and cytoplasmic viscosity. Alterations in their structure and properties cause impairments in functioning and reduce survival. This chapter focusses on the causes of these modifications and their clinical implications. Erythrocyte disorders can be broadly divided into the following categories:

1. Membrane disorders: Variations in the structure of the membrane and shape of RBCs can be due to:
   - Skeletal defects reduce mechanical resistance and lifespan (hereditary spherocytosis, hereditary elliptosis, hereditary pyropoikilocytosis and South Asian ovalocytosis)
   - Changes in cation permeability and transport reduces osmotic resistance (hereditary stomatocytosis)
   - Other causes - oxidative stress and increase in calcium levels
2. Hemoglobinopathies: Disorders due to globin gene mutations such as sickle cell disease and thalassemia also cause secondary effects.
3. Volume homeostasis:
   - Primary disorders include inherent disorders of volume regulation (hereditary xerocytosis)
   - Secondary diseases due to other RBC disorders
4. Oxidative stress:
   - Production of reactive species in RBCs, which directly leads to protein oxidation and lipid peroxidation
   - Other acute and chronic diseases such as cardiovascular diseases, malaria, liver disease, etc.
5. Metabolic disorders or Enzymopathies: Defects in enzymes related to:
   - Glycolysis - pyruvate kinase, hexokinase, aldolase, etc.
   - Hexose monophosphate shunt - glucose-6-phosphate dehydrogenase, glutathione peroxidase, etc.
   - Other enzyme deficiencies - pyrimidine-5'-nucleotidase, ATPase, etc.

These disorders, either as primary causes or in association with other conditions, clinically manifest into anemia and its related ailments. Anemia is triggered by blood loss, surge in erythrocyte destruction or impairment in their production and also by variations in erythrocyte shape, size and hemoglobin content. Supplementation of iron, folic acid and vitamin B_{12} are used to treat mild cases of anemia, while RBC transfusions are preferred in severe cases. Transfusions are the primary interventions employed to subside the severity of erythrocyte disorders. Better blood banking and increased availability of blood would provide far reaching effects into the treatment of erythrocyte disorders.

Keywords: erythrocyte disorders, hemoglobinopathies, enzymopathies, membrane disorders

INTRODUCTION

Erythrocytes or red blood cells (RBC) are a predominant cellular component of blood, mainly responsible for the transport of respiratory gases (oxygen and carbon dioxide). They are biconcave disc shaped structures measuring 7.2 to 7.8μm in diameter with a thickness of 1μm in the center and 2μm at the periphery. These cells contain a cytoplasm-devoid of nuclei and major organelles, surrounded by a fluid plasma membrane.

Erythrocytes are produced by "erythropoiesis," which is a systematic cycle of formation of erythrocytes from stem cells in the bone marrow. Pluripotent hematopoietic stem cells undergo differentiation into committed myeloid cells which can produce all the blood cells. These myeloid series differentiate into erythrocyte producing progenitor cells known as "colony forming units-erythrocytes (CFU-E) which yield proerythroblasts/pronormoblasts. Proerythroblasts are characterized by large nuclei, devoid of hemoglobin and measure 15 to 20μm. These precursors show decreases in size, condensation of nuclei and accumulation of hemoglobin & eosinophilic cytoplasm, through differentiation involving basophil, polychromatophil and orthochromatic erythroblasts. Finally, reticulocytes are formed after 6 days of differentiation from proerythroblasts, by dissolving of the nucleus, reabsorption of endoplasmic reticulum and abundance of hemoglobin & remnants of cytoplasmic organelles. These cells enter the blood stream and lose the remaining organelles and basophilic materials, forming the mature erythrocyte in 1-2 days. The process of erythropoiesis is regulated by various hematopoietic growth factors, mainly erythropoietin, which stimulates the formation of proerythroblasts from the CFU-E. The maturation of erythrocytes also requires vitamin B_{12} (cyanocobalamin) and folic acid, which assist in cell differentiation. Mature erythrocytes last for a period of 120 days in circulation, following which they are destroyed in the spleen [1, 2].

Hemoglobin (Hb) is the main erythrocyte constituent which is an iron-containing protein, responsible for carrying oxygen to tissues and acting as a blood buffer. Hemoglobin is made up of "heme"- an iron containing compound, belonging to the protoporphyrin group, and "globin"- a protein containing four polypeptide chains. The affinity of the heme group to oxygen and binding of oxygen to the iron in heme accounts for the oxygen carrying capacity of erythrocytes, and thereby their effective functioning. Hemoglobin is degraded during senescence into iron and globin, of which the heme is converted into biliverdin. The iron is converted into ferritin, which is stored and later recycled into hemoglobin.

Erythrocyte membrane is responsible for the antigenic, transport and mechanical properties [3], characterized by a semipermeable asymmetric lipid bilayer, supported by a mesh-like cytoskeleton [4-6]. The lipid bilayer is interspersed with internal hydrophilic peripheral proteins, middle hydrophobic integral proteins (mainly band 3 and glycophorins) and external hydrophilic proteins. The glycophorins at the outer surface possess an NH_2-terminal to which the blood group antigens, ABO and MN attach, while the inner COOH domain faces the cytoplasm and interacts with the cytoskeleton [7-10]. Band 3 is the most abundant protein in the erythrocyte membrane [11], consisting of an anion exchange channel (exchange of bicarbonate and chloride ions), assisting in membrane stability and facilitating erythrocyte removal during senescence [12]. Band 3 provides membrane crosslinking through association of the lipid bilayer to the cytoskeleton [13, 14].

The cytoskeleton comprises of some major peripheral proteins which are spectrin, ankyrin, actin and Band 4.1R. Spectrin facilitates the formation of a complex intracellular network by (i) interactions of spectrin-actin-Band 4.1R junction complexes with the cytoplasmic domain of glycophorin (horizontal interactions) and (ii) binding to ankyrin, which consecutively binds to the cytoplasmic domain of Band 3 via Band 4.2 (vertical interactions). The structural organization of the erythrocyte membrane plays a major role in RBC functioning, increases the surface area for diffusion and enables deformability.

Erythrocytes rely on anaerobic metabolic pathways to produce energy, consisting primarily of glycolysis and three secondary pathways- pentose phosphate pathway, methemoglobin reductase pathway and the Rapoport-Leubering shunt. These pathways allow for the formation of an allosteric inhibitor of hemoglobin, known as 2,3-diphosphoglycerate, lactic acid and ATP, while maintaining heme in the reduced state.

Erythrocytes are very well suited to carry out their functions due to: (i) a dynamic cell membrane, (ii) cell geometry, i.e., the inherent shape and lack of organelles and (iii) cytoplasmic viscosity maintained by the presence of hemoglobin [3]. However, any alterations in membrane, cell geometry, deformability, flow properties and increases in cell viscosity directly influence erythrocyte functioning and survival. The causes of these variations are discussed in detail in this chapter and can be grouped as follows (Figure 1):

1. Membrane Disorders
2. Hemoglobinopathies
3. Volume Homeostasis
4. Oxidative Stress
5. Metabolic Disorders/Enzymopathies

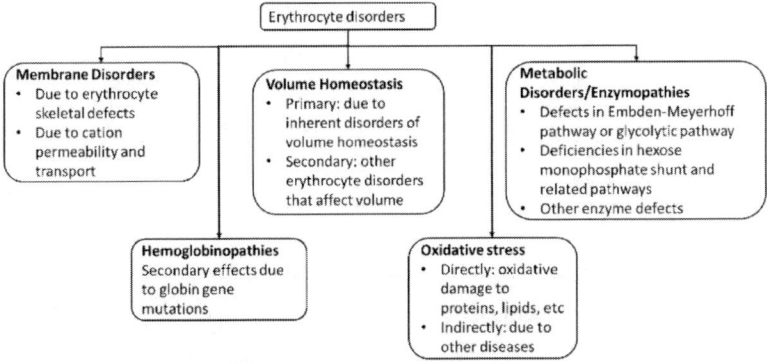

Figure 1. Schematic representation of erythrocyte disorders.

MEMBRANE DISORDERS

Modifications or variations in the structural components of the erythrocyte membrane and the interactions between these components directly affect the functional integrity of the membrane. The interactions between membrane components, specifically the membrane proteins may be vertical (between lipid bilayer and cytoskeleton: involving band 3, spectrin, ankyrin and band 4.2) or horizontal (between constituents of the cytoskeletal network: involving spectrin, band 4.1 and ankyrin) [15]. The vertical interactions aid erythrocyte membrane cohesion, while the horizontal or lateral interactions aid erythrocyte mechanical stability [5]. The maintenance of cohesion and stability, in turn are crucial for preserving erythrocyte shape, surface area and deformability [5]. Therefore, any modifications in the RBC membrane proteins directly lead to loss of surface area, deformability, reduction of lifespan and hence hemolytic anemia. These hereditary disorders [16] may be classified as those due to (a) mutations in membrane or skeletal proteins or (b) defects in cation permeability and transport [17].

MUTATIONS IN MEMBRANE AND SKELETAL PROTEINS

These changes cause decreases in mechanical resistance of red cells and hence directly reduce lifespan [17].

Defects in Vertical Interactions

Reductions in spectrin density causes loss of cohesion between the cytoskeleton and lipid bilayer, while deficiencies in band 3, ankyrin and band 4.2 reduce the number of linkages between the bilayer and cytoskeleton [18]. Both these types of variations cause hereditary spherocytosis (HS).

Hereditary spherocytosis shows high prevalence in the Caucasian and Japanese populations [19], affecting 1 out of every 2,000-3,000 individuals making it the most common hereditary red cell membrane disorder [20], following an autosomal dominant inheritance pattern [21] in 75% of cases [3, 20]. This disease is caused due to genetic modifications or molecular defects in ankyrin (*ANK1* gene), spectrin (*SPTA1* and *SPTB* genes), band 3 (*SLC4A1* gene) and protein 4.2 (*EPB42* gene), where defects in *ANK1* gene is most prevalent [5, 16-17, 19-20]. The disease is characterized by spherical erythrocytes in the peripheral blood smear [16] in contrast to the normal biconcave shape of erythrocytes. They also contain larger amounts of hemoglobin [19] and lose membrane by vesiculation, thereby reducing surface area [18] and are eventually phagocytosed causing hemolytic anemia [22]. The symptoms of this disease also include jaundice, reticulocytosis, gallstones and splenomegaly [5].

Defects in Horizontal or Lateral Interactions (Hereditary)

Any defects in the dimerization of spectrin and in between the interactions of spectrin, actin and protein 4.1R, account for loss of membrane stability and the prevalence of hereditary elliptocytosis (HE) and its related disorders.

   a. *Hereditary Elliptocytosis (HE):* This acquired disorder has a prevalence of 1 out of every 2,000-4,000 individuals [16, 20], but shows higher prevalence in West African countries, which are endemic to malaria [5, 16, 23]. The disorder usually follows an autosomal dominant pattern of inheritance [20] and is caused mainly due to defects in spectrin (*SPTA1* and *SPTB* genes) and protein 4.1 (*EPB41* gene) [19]. Due to these molecular defects, the erythrocytes are elliptically shaped or elongated, which could be asymptomatic or show severe hemolytic anemia [19, 24].
   b. *Hereditary Pyropoikilocytosis (HPP)* is a severe symptomatic manifestation of HE [17], where the erythrocytes are abnormally shaped, resembling the erythrocytes which have been exposed to high

temperatures or a thermal burn [5, 25]. These erythrocytes also show abnormal osmotic fragility and hence show losses of mechanical resistance and surface area [16].

c. *South Asian Ovalocytosis (SAO)* is a unique manifestation of elliptosis, characterized by oval-shaped erythrocytes with one or two longitudinal slits [5, 16]. This disorder is named after its prevalence in the South East Asian countries, that it is most prevalent in such as, Indonesia, Philippines, Thailand, Papua New Guinea and Malaysia [5, 16-17, 26-27]. Although this disorder may be asymptomatic, it follows an autosomal dominant type of inheritance and is due to a deletion in *SCL4A1* gene of band 3, thereby causing increased rigidity and decreased deformability in the affected erythrocytes [17, 28].

These hereditary elliptocytosis and their associated disorders, show a wide range of phenotypes from mild to severe hemolytic anemia. However, their prevalence in malaria endemic countries are high, as these disorders provide some natural immunity against malaria, as the rigidity of the erythrocyte membrane prevents infection by the malarial parasite [16, 28].

DEFECTS IN CATION PERMEABILITY AND TRANSPORT

These defects cause reductions in osmotic resistance and are due to defects in Na^+ and K^+ transport. These disorders are also known as leaky membrane syndromes [17] and constitute a group of disorders known as hereditary stomatocytosis (HSt).

Hereditary stomatocytosis is characterized by the presence of stomata shaped or mouth-shaped stoma in the center of the cell [16] or are said to be "bowl-shaped" [29]. The modifications in cation permeability and ion transport have a direct effect on the volume and hence the surface area to volume ratio of the erythrocytes, thereby hampering their functioning and eventually, their lifespan [5]. Increase in the erythrocyte volume is known as hydrocytosis, while a decrease is known as xerocytosis [16]. The disorder shows varied symptomatic syndromes and can be classified as:

Overhydrated HSt, Dehydrated HSt (xerocytosis), Cryohydrocytosis and Familial pseudohyperkalemia (FP)[20]. Stomatocytosis shows varied symptomatic phenotypes, whose molecular causes are not yet very clearly understood [5, 16, 30-31], showing mutations in stomatin, band 3, flotillin, *PIEZO1*, etc.

   a. *Overhydrated HSt:* In this form of stomatocytosis, erythrocytes show an increase in volume, hemolysis and osmotic fragility [5, 16]. These erythrocytes show high sodium ion levels, thereby elevating water content of the cell and hence its volume [16]. Higher cell volume in turn reduces mean corpuscular hemoglobin concentration (MCHC) without changes in surface area [5] and consequently results in cells which are osmotically fragile [16]. This disorder follows an autosomal dominant inheritance pattern [5].
   b. *Dehydrated HSt:* This form of stomatocytosis is characterized by xerocytosis or dehydrated, contracted erythrocytes [16] and is inherited in an autosomal dominant manner [5]. The xerocytosis phenotype i.e., decrease in cell volume, causes increase in mean corpuscular Hb concentration and concomitant increase in osmotic fragility, leading to anemia [5]. The erythrocytes are unable to regulate cation homeostasis [3], show lower levels of ions (sodium and potassium) within the erythrocytes, leading to loss of water from the cell cytoplasm [29]. This disorder occurs more frequently than OHSt, but is less frequent than HS [17, 29], sometimes found to be caused by mutations in *PIEZO1* (a mechanotransduction protein) [32].
   c. *Cryohydrocytosis:* This disorder is a variation from DHSt and OHSt as it is shows hemolysis and high cell volume only when the cells are stored at low temperatures [29]. The genetic aspects of this disease are however yet to be proven and hence this disorder is usually assumed to be a part of OHSt [17].
   d. *Familial pseudohyperkalemia:* This syndrome can occur independently or in association with the other stomatocytosis disorders. This disorder of cation homeostasis is rare, as it is often overlooked due to its normal hematology. However, a test for

potassium levels after standing for a few hours can be utilized in diagnosis, as the results show a raised plasma potassium level [29].

HEMOGLOBINOPATHIES

The main function of erythrocytes is to transport oxygen via hemoglobin. Hence, any modifications or defects in hemoglobin itself can play a major role in the efficient functioning of the erythrocyte. The damage to hemoglobin can occur due to genetic defects or due to oxidative stress. The causes and effects of oxidative damage on hemoglobin and hence its effects on the erythrocyte membrane will be discussed in the following section on Oxidative stress.

Hemoglobinopathies, usually include disorders and syndromes arising from inherited abnormalities in the globin gene. *"Hereditary disorders of hemoglobin can be broadly classified into those which result from defects in biosynthetic mechanisms, with resultant quantitative alterations in the amount of the affected subunit of hemoglobin, which is qualitatively normal, or in alterations in the structure of a subunit to yield a qualitatively abnormal hemoglobin,"* as stated by Ramney and Lehmann [33]. The latter group, constitutes a variety of syndromes, together known as the thalassemia syndromes.

Hemoglobin is mainly made up of two pairs of non-alike globin chains, most commonly α and β, however, γ and δ chains are also observed in fetal and some adult hemoglobins, respectively [34]. Normal adult hemoglobin consists of two α and two β globin chains, commonly denoted as $\alpha_2\beta_2$ hemoglobin or HbA [34]. Structural alterations or modifications in hemoglobin occur due to amino acid substitutions, deletions, non-homologous or unequal crossing-over and polypeptide chain elongation [33].

Sickle Cell Disease (SCD)

This disease usually represents a group of disorders which show a sickle cell shaped erythrocyte morphology, caused due to the presence of homozygous sickle-cell hemoglobin (HbS). This involves a missense substitution of valine instead of glutamic acid, leading to this abnormal β chain hemoglobin [35, 36]. HbS, unlike normal hemoglobin, has a low affinity for oxygen, causing polymerization of the HbS at low oxygen concentrations, leading to change in shape of erythrocytes, from biconcave discs, to elongated, sickle shaped cells, consequently decreasing erythrocyte deformability [35, 37]. This leads to loss of erythrocyte functioning and finally anemia, as these cells begin to hemolyze and be rapidly removed from the body. SCD affects the cardiothoracic system (chronic restrictive lung disease, left ventricular diastolic disease, pulmonary hypertension, dysrhythmias and acute chest syndrome), nervous system (hemorrhagic stroke, acute ischemic stroke, silent cerebral infarctions, venous sinus thrombosis, proliferative retinopathy, orbital infarction and chronic pain in limbs), reticuloendothelial system (splenic sequestration and functional hyposplenism), gastrointestinal system (hepatopathy, cholangiopathy, cholelithiasis and mesenteric vaso-occlusion), urogenital system (papillary necrosis, proteinuria, renal failure, hematuria, nocturnal enuresis and priapism) and musculoskeletal system (avascular necrosis and leg ulcerations) [38-39]. The sickle cell disease syndromes consist of sickle cell anemia (SCA), HbSC (HbS and HbC- where glutamic acid is substituted with lysine) and HBSβ-thalassemia (explained in thalassemia section), all formed due to mutations in the *Hbβ* gene [35]. SCD shows an incidence of 300,000 individuals per year [40], of which SCA, the most prevalent form of SCD constitutes about 75% [40], observed predominantly in sub-Saharan Africa [35]. SCA follows a recessive mode of inheritance, hence only individuals with both β-genes affected show clear symptoms of the disease. Although SCA is due to mutations in Hbβ, the symptoms and severity of the disease varies among individuals, however, the most common binding feature of all patients with SCA, is chronic hemolytic anemia [35]. HbSC, is also most commonly found in African countries, and this genotype for hemoglobin shows a certain resistance against malaria [34]. The HbCC genotype is also observed in the same geographical area, showing milder symptoms of SCA [34].

Thalassemias

Thalassemias are a group of inherited disorders where there is a reduction or absence in the production of the globin chain [41], found in the Mediterranean and South East Asian regions of the world [34]. In these syndromes, no structural abnormality is observed in the globin chain, however the quantity of the protein is diminished or absent [42], causing abnormal functioning and flattened shape of erythrocytes [34]. These disorders show a wide range of symptoms, which depend on (i) the polypeptide chain that is affected (α and β mainly), (ii) the inherited pattern (homozygous or heterozygous) and (iii) reduction or absence of the polypeptide chain [34].

α-Thalassemia is observed when one or two (of the four α-genes for *Hbα*) are deleted. This accordingly leads to α^+(-α/αα) or α^o (--/αα) genotypes, which does not show very prominent symptoms [37] but can be a genetic modifier in case of sickle cell disease [36]. The absence of three out of the four α genes causes a rare and unique disease known as Hemoglobin H, prevalent in South East Asia, which shows severe anemic symptoms [37]. The absence of all four α-genes produces a syndrome known as Hemoglobin Bart's *hydrops fetalis*, where in most cases, the infant does not survive due to complete lack of *Hbα* [37].

β-Thalassemia is observed as genotypes like α-thalassemia but is due to deletions in the *Hbβ* genes of hemoglobin. The heterozygous forms of this disorder (e.g., $\beta^S\beta^+$: HbS with a Hbβ deletion), usually shows mild symptoms of anemia (similar to SCA) and is known as thalassemia minor [34, 37]. The serious and severe form of the disease is evident when a homozygous condition is observed, where symptoms are severe with hemolytic anemia and splenomegaly [33].

VOLUME HOMEOSTASIS

Any modifications in erythrocyte volume, due to direct or indirect causes, leads to variations in the efficient functioning of erythrocytes, deformability and osmotic fragility. These modifications in volume or in the control of volume homeostasis, can be inherited or due to repercussions of other erythrocyte disorders [43]. The primary inherited disorders of volume homeostasis overlap with the genetic defects in cation permeability and transport, collectively the hereditary stomatocytosis syndromes, as discussed earlier inthsi chapter. The secondary disorders that influence changes in erythrocyte volume are hereditary spherocytosis, thalassemia and sickle cell syndromes and even malaria [44]. A unique abnormality in the glucose transporter protein in erythrocytes (GLUT1), leading to cation leaks and symptoms similar to stomatocytosis, has also been found to be a secondary cause of abnormalities in maintenance of erythrocyte volume [44].

OXIDATIVE STRESS

Oxidative stress is defined as, *"a disturbance in the prooxdiant-antioxidant balance in favor of the former, leading to potential damage"* [45]. Modifications in hemoglobin, proteins and lipids due to the action of reactive oxygen species (ROS), constitutes and results in oxidative damage in erythrocytes.

Changes in hemoglobin due to oxidative stress can directly lead to membrane injury and these changes are mainly due to autooxidation of hemoglobin. The formation of methemoglobin can occur by the loss of a superoxide anion from oxyhemoglobin, containing oxidized iron (Fe^{3+}) [46-47]. This reaction initiates the formation and conversion of different reactive oxygen species, which cause oxidative stress and consequently, oxidative damage. The methemoglobin produced can be modified by hydrogen peroxide (H_2O_2) into oxoferryl Hb, which in turn reacts with oxygen to form irreversible sulfhemoglobin and choleglobin [48] and peroxyl radicals. Hydrogen peroxide mediates reactions between methemoglobin and lipids, hence causing further oxidative damage [49]. The irreversible choleglobin and sulfhemoglobin bind to lipids, mainly phosphatidylserine in the membrane, thereby disrupting erythrocyte shape [49]. There is evidence to show that Hb binds to the membrane and cytoskeleton during increased oxidative stress [50], interacting with spectrin, band 3, ankyrin and band 4.2 [51].

The formation of superoxide radicals by autooxidation of Hb is one of the primary steps that cause production of other reactive species [52]. Superoxides can produce potent hydroxyl radicals via Fenton and Haber-Weiss reactions as erythrocytes contain large amounts of iron which catalyze these reactions [45]. Superoxides also react with nitric oxide to form peroxynitrite radicals [53]. This ROS cascade damages proteins and lipids of erythrocytes, mainly in the membrane.

The predominance of polyunsaturated fatty acids and an oxygen abundant environment increases the susceptibility of erythrocytes to lipid peroxidation and the formation of various products of lipid peroxidation. The short-lived, intermediate primary products are known as conjugate dienes and are formed during propagation of lipid peroxidation. These further react with ROS to form peroxyl radicals which continue the peroxidation process and produce secondary products such as malondialdehyde, isoprostanes, 4-hydroxynonenal, etc. [54]. These products subsequently react with other products of protein oxidation and lipid peroxidation, causing further damage to erythrocytes. Malondialdehyde is a prominent lipid peroxidation product that causes crosslinking of other proteins and lipids, leading to loss of anion transport and function of Band 3 [50, 52, 55]. The exposure of phosphatidylserine and peroxidation of lipids contribute to the loss of membrane via microvesicles, in turn leading to irreversible damage of the erythrocyte membrane [56-57].

Protein oxidation is defined as *"the covalent modification of a protein induced either directly by ROS or indirectly by reaction with secondary by-products of oxidative stress"* [58]. Damage to proteins occur by both radical (superoxide, hydroxyl, peroxyl, alkoxyl and hydroperoxyl) and non-radical species (hydrogen peroxide and hypochlorous acid) [59]. Various products of protein oxidation may occur based on the site of attack by ROS, i.e., the backbone (causing breakage, protein-protein and protein-lipid interactions) or side chains (protein carbonyls) [60]. The interactions between protein and lipid products of oxidation lead to the formation of advanced lipoxidation or glycation end products [59]. Sulfhydryls maintain cellular integrity, maintain redox balance and provide mechanical strength. Glutathione and band 3 consist of protein sulfhydryl groups, which upon oxidation can be reversibly or irreversibly damaged [61]. Protein cross-linking products due to dityrosine linkages, characterized as advanced oxidation protein products (AOPP) [62] are also formed. The abnormal binding of spectrin-actin-Band 4.1R and the oxidative damage to Band 3 also creates neo-antigens that lead to antibody-mediated RBC clearance [55]. Protein oxidation and lipid peroxidation lead to loss of membrane integrity, microvesicle formation, hemolysis and apoptosis.

Oxidative stress can also be induced in Alzheimer's, liver disease, malaria, hypertension, cancer, diabetes, cardiovascular disease, chronic obstructive pulmonary disorder, etc. The interrelation between oxidative stress and these disorders has been well established [63-66], which can be characterized as secondary causes of erythrocyte modifications.

METABOLIC DISORDERS/ENZYMOPATHIES

Mature erythrocytes do not possess mitochondria and ribosomes; however, they demonstrate a complex active metabolism, which sustains their structure and function [67-68]. They rely on anaerobic metabolic pathways for energy and maintenance of homeostasis. The metabolic pathways can be grouped into (i) glycolysis and related metabolic pathways, (ii) antioxidant pathways (for synthesis of available antioxidants and maintaining iron in Hb in reduced state) and (iii) nucleotide metabolism. Since these are usually interconnected and interrelated, any aberration in the enzymes involved has a direct influence on erythrocyte function, mainly causing a range of hemolytic anemias. However, in order to understand the enzymopathies of erythrocytes which play important roles phenotypically, the disorders can be grouped as depicted in Figure 2.

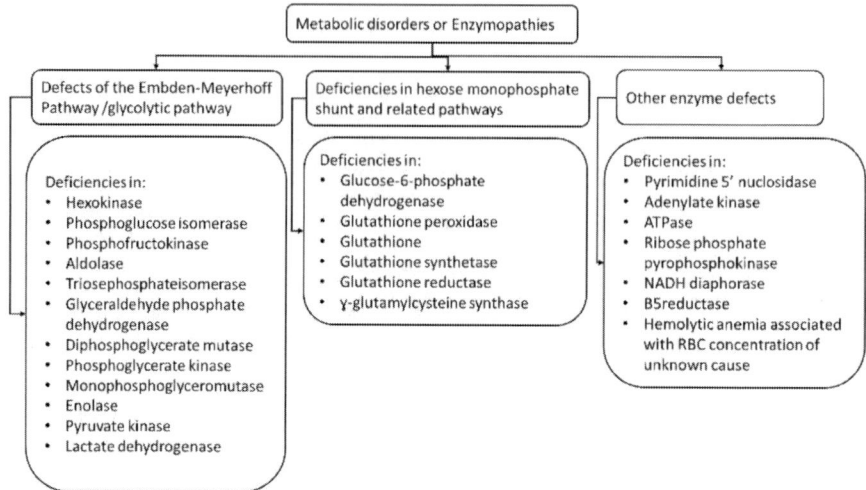

Figure 2. Schematic representation of metabolic disorders of erythrocytes [68-69, 73].

DEFECTS OF EMDEN-MEYERHOFF PATHWAY/GLYCOLYTIC PATHWAY

Erythrocytes depend on glycolysis as their primary source of energy and as the basis for other metabolic pathways. The enzymes related to the glycolytic pathway, whose deficiency causes an erythrocyte disorder are depicted in Figure 2. These enzyme defects and deficiencies usually follow an autosomal recessive pattern of inheritance and show a clear phenotype with non-spherocytic congenital hemolytic anemia [69].

- *Hexokinase (HK):* This enzyme phosphorylates glucose to glucose-6 phosphate in the first step of glycolysis and is encoded by the *HK-1* gene. This deficiency is rare and follows an autosomal recessive pattern [69-70], reported in 17-19 families worldwide [68, 71]. This enzyme is considered as one of the rate-limiting enzymes in glycolysis [70-71], as it possesses the least activity [68] among all glycolytic enzymes.

- *Phosphoglucose isomerase (PGI) or Glucose phosphate isomerase (GPI):* Deficiency in this enzyme is the second most common glycolytic enzyme deficiency [72] after pyruvate kinase, following an autosomal recessive inheritance pattern [67, 73] and reported in 50-100 families worldwide [71, 74]. This enzyme facilitates the interconversion of glucose-6-phosphate and fructose-6-phosphate, in the second step of glycolysis. The deficiency of GPI is attributed to mutations in the *GPI* gene, causing loss of reverse isomerization of fructose-6-phosphate to glucose-6-phosphate and thereby loss of conversion of fructose-6-phosphate (also produced by the hexose monophosphate shunt) [67, 75].
- *Phosphofructokinase (PFK):* This enzyme catalyzes the conversion of fructose-6-phosphate to fructose-1,6-biphsophate. Mutations in the *PFK-M* gene, found in 30 families (Ashkenazi Jews [68]) have been attributed to deficiency in PFK enzyme [76].
- *Aldolase:* Conversion of fructose-1,6-biphosphate into glyceraldehyde-3-phosphate and dihydroxyacetone phosphate is catalyzed by aldolase. Mutations in *ALDOA* gene have been reported in 6-10 patients from five families [77], however, this deficiency is extremely rare [68]. The defect in aldolase gene also affects hereditary spherocytosis [69].
- *Triosephosphate isomerase (TPI):* This enzyme shows the highest activity among all the glycolytic enzymes [78] and is utilized in the catalysis of glyceraldehyde-3-phosphate and dihydroxyacetone phosphate. Mutations in the *TPI1* gene leads to deficiency of TPI enzyme. The most common mutation is a substitution of aspartic acid at a site for glutamic acid (occurring 74% of the time) [68, 79-80].
- *Diphosphoglycerate mutase or bisphosphoglycerate mutase (BPGM):* This enzyme plays a crucial role in the efficient functioning of erythrocytes. It catalyzes the conversion of 1,3-diphosphoglycerate to 2,3-diphosphoglycerate, which is an allosteric binder to Hb facilitating dissociation of oxygen from Hb [69]. The 2,3-

diphosphoglycerate is then converted by this enzyme into 3-phosphoglycerate, thereby regulating the levels of 2,3-diphosphoglycerate [68].

- *Phosphoglycerate kinase (PGK):* This enzyme assists in the interconversion of 1,3-biphosphoglycerate and 3-biphosphoglycerate, with the production of one molecule of ATP [68-69, 71]. Mutations in the *PGK1* gene (16 mutations [81]) cause deficiencies in this enzyme and this disorder follows an X-linked inheritance pattern [82]. However as this reaction can be bypassed by the Rapoport-Leubering shunt, very few cases are observed [68].
- *Monophosphoglyceromutase (MPGM):* Found in only one case, attributed to an abnormal B subunit of the enzyme, caused due to a mutation in the *MPGM* gene [83-84]. This enzyme assists in the reversible reaction of converting 3-phosphoglyceric acid to 2-phosphoglyceric acid, utilizing 2,3-diphosphoglycerate as an intermediate.
- *Enolase:* This enzyme converts 2-phosphoglyceric acid to phosphoenol pyruvate but does not clearly show any phenotypic symptoms of anemia [69].
- *Pyruvate kinase (PK):* Deficiency in pyruvate kinase is the most prevalent enzyme deficiency of glycolysis [85] accounting for more than 90% of all glycolytic enzyme deficiencies [86]. It is common in Northern Europe [87-88] and has a prevalence of 1 in 20,000 [37, 68, 89]. It is an autosomal recessive disorder and the most common cause of hereditary non-spherocytic anemia [75, 90]. This enzyme is involved in production of ATP during the dephosphorylation of phosphoenol pyruvate to pyruvic acid. Hence, defects in this enzyme cause reduction in utilizing glucose, loss of ATP production [68, 73], abnormal membrane functioning with loss of potassium and water, leading to hemolysis [85]. Mutations in *PKLR* gene cause deficiency of pyruvate kinase enzyme and over 200 mutations in this gene have been discovered [67-68, 73].
- *Lactate dehydrogenase (LDH):* Although modifications in the subunits of LDH enzyme have been reported, no phenotypic symptoms have been observed in the deficiency of this enzyme [91-

92]. This enzyme is responsible for maintaining the equilibrium between lactate and pyruvate in erythrocytes [69]. It follows an autosomal recessive type of inheritance pattern [69].

DEFICIENCIES IN HEXOSE MONOPHOSPHATE SHUNT AND RELATED PATHWAYS

These deficiencies are characterized in enzymes that are involved in the hexose-monophosphate or Rapoport-Leubering shunt and their related metabolic pathways, such as glutathione synthesis. These deficiencies show some similarities to those of the glycolytic pathway and intensify during oxidative stress [69].

- *Glucose-6-phosphate dehydrogenase (G6PD):* This enzyme is the primary enzyme in the hexose monophosphate shunt, catalyzing the conversion of glucose-6-phosphate to 6-phosphogluconate, involving the reduction of NADP to NADPH. This reduction via the shunt is a significant step in protecting erythrocytes from oxidative stress [90] and is important in maintaining glutathione in its reduced state [73]. The deficiency of this enzyme is the most prevalent erythrocyte enzymopathy, observed usually in malaria endemic regions [68], such as in Mediterranean, Asian and African populations. It affects 400-500 million people [68, 73] and is inherited as a X-linked disorder [69, 90]. Many variants of this disorder (greater than 400 [68]) have been reported, mainly with mutations in the *G6PD* gene [90], leading to a wide variety of phenotypes, ranging from mild to severe G6PD deficiency [67]. The most common deficiencies are in G6PDA (found predominantly in Africa) and G6PD-Mediterranean isoforms (prevalent in the Mediterranean region) [68]. The disorder is characterized by loss of deformability, high osmotic fragility and elevated hemolysis [73]. The varying phenotypes show acute and chronic hemolysis, favism, neonatal jaundice, etc [68].
- *Glutathione peroxidase (GSH-Px):* The antioxidant defenses of erythrocytes include enzymatic components such as GSH-Px and non-

enzymatic components, such as glutathione. This enzyme causes the breakdown or degradation of H_2O_2, utilizing glutathione as a substrate [69] and oxidizing glutathione [75]. Hence, reduction or deficiency in this enzyme will directly reduce the antioxidant capacity of the erythrocytes [93].

- *Glutathione (GSH):* Glutathione is a non-enzymatic antioxidant, commonly found in erythrocytes. It is a tripeptide made up of glutamic acid, cysteine and glycine and its deficiency is inherited as an autosomal recessive disorder [69].
- *Glutathione reductase (GR):* This enzyme is responsible for the reduction of oxidized glutathione (GSSG) back into glutathione, which is necessary for protecting erythrocytes from oxidative damage [68]. This deficiency is caused a by a large deletion in the *GR* gene, leading to mild anemia and jaundice [68].
- *Glutathione synthetase (GS):* The second step of glutathione synthesis, i.e., the condensation of γ-glutamylcysteine and glycine is catalyzed by this enzyme [68]. Deficiency of this enzyme leads to an accumulation of 5-oxoproline (a metabolite of γ-glutamylcysteine), which causes hemolysis and neurological defects [68].
- *γ-glutamylcysteine synthase:* This enzyme is responsible for the catalysis of the initial step of glutathione synthesis, whose deficiency is rare, with symptoms of hemolytic anemia and neurological defects [68].

OTHER ENZYME DEFECTS

Modifications in enzymes involved in other metabolic pathways, occasionally play a role in the formation of enzymopathies [69].

- *Pyrimidine 5' nucleosidase (P5'N):* The deficiency of this enzyme is the third most prevalent erythrocyte enzymopathy [67-68]. This enzyme catalyzes the conversion of nucleotides (cytidine and uridine) to nucleosides which can diffuse through the erythrocytes [72, 94]. Hence, a deficiency in this enzyme leads to accumulation of nucleotides in the erythrocytes causing hemolysis [68]. This is an autosomal recessive, rare erythrocyte disorder [71, 73], which causes chronic hemolytic anemia [68].

- *NADH diaphorase:* This enzyme is also known as NADH-dependent methemoglobin reductase enzyme. This enzyme is crucial in the conversion of methemoglobin back into hemoglobin, with the oxidation of NADPH. The deficiency of this enzyme is observed in patients as one of the major causes of methemoglobinemia [69].

- *B5reductase (B5R):* A deficiency in B5reductases, leads to a condition known as hereditary methemoglobinemia [67-68]. This deficiency occurs due to mutations in the cytochrome b5 reductase enzyme, leading to type I and type II methemoglobinemia [95]. These types are based on the clinical severity of the disease, where type I is a milder form showing only cyanosis, while type II, the severe form shows cyanosis associated with mental retardation, slowed growth and death prior to puberty [67]. These deficiencies are inherited in an autosomal recessive manner, leading to congenital methemoglobinemia [68].

CONSEQUENCES OF ERYTHROCYTE DISORDERS

It is evident that almost all disorders of erythrocytes, irrespective of their cause, show a phenotypic characteristic of some form of anemia. *"Anemia is a condition in which the red blood cells are reduced in number or volume or are deficient in hemoglobin,"* as stated by Kara Rogers [34]. Anemia is mainly caused due to (i) abnormalities in erythrocyte production, (ii) increased hemolysis (reduced erythrocyte survival), (iii) accumulation of normal erythrocytes in spleen and (iv) degradation of abnormal erythrocytes [96].

A schematic representation of anemia and its types based on etiology and pathogenesis is depicted in Figure 3a., while the types of anemia based on erythrocyte size, shape and hemoglobin content is depicted in Figure 3b.

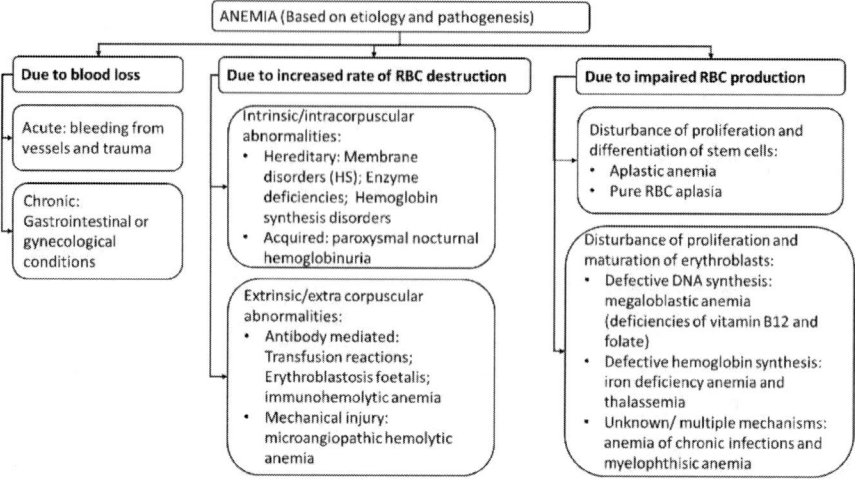

Figure 3a. Anemia (based on etiology and pathogenesis) [34, 96-97].

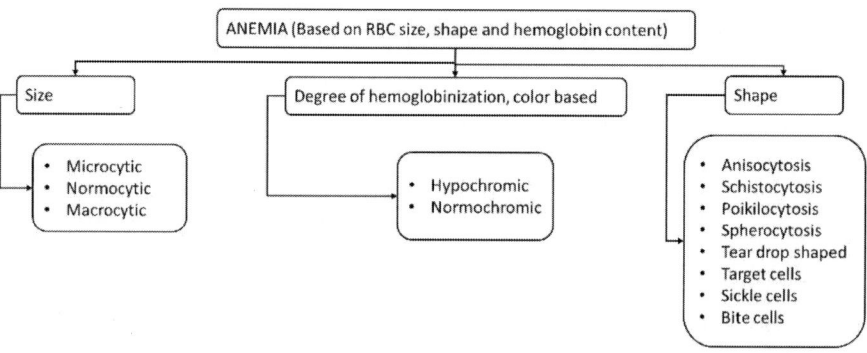

Figure 3b. Anemia (based on erythrocyte size, shape and hemoglobin content) [34, 96-97].

Diagnosis and Treatment of Erythrocyte Disorders

Most erythrocyte disorders are initially diagnosed based on a peripheral blood smear, erythrocyte counts, indices, morphology [97] and hemolytic properties. The lack of a well-defined cause deduced from the blood smear and tests for hemolysis, subsequently requires the use of more sophisticated and specific tools and tests to diagnose an erythrocyte disorder. The determination of the type of erythrocyte disorder is imperative to pave way for the appropriate treatment and management strategies. Mild anemia is usually treated with supplementation of iron, folic acid and vitamin B_{12}. Erythrocyte disorders, their diagnoses and treatment are outlined in Table 1.

Table 1. Erythrocyte disorders: diagnosis and treatment

Erythrocyte disorder	Diagnosis methods	Treatments/Management	Ref
Membrane defects	Blood smear, osmotic fragility	Splenectomy and transfusions	[16]
Sickle cell anemia	Electrophoresis and High-performance liquid chromatography (HPLC) of hemoglobin	Hydroxycarbamide, RBC transfusions and hematopoietic stem cell transplantations	[35]
Due to Oxidative stress	Protein, lipid and hemoglobin oxidation products, hemolysis	Antioxidant supplementation	[93]
G6PD deficiency	Rapid fluorescent screening test or by quantitative spectrophotometric analysis	Folate supplementation and blood transfusions	[68]
B5reductase deficiency	Cyanosis Spectrophotometric methemoglobin estimation	Methylene blue and ascorbic acid	[68]
Pyruvate kinase deficiency	Crude hemolysate test, low enzyme levels	RBC transfusions and in severe cases, splenectomy	[68, 73]
Pyrimidine 5'nucleosidase deficiency	Presence of nucleosides in RBC	Chronic transfusions and splenectomy	[68]
Glutathione synthetase deficiency	Presence of 5-oxoproline	Correction of metabolic acidosis and antioxidant supplementation	[68]

CONCLUSION

Erythrocytes are crucial in the effective functioning of the human body as they provide oxygen for all cellular processes. Defects, modifications and disorders of erythrocytes have a wide range of causes ranging from genetic to oxidative damage. The survival of erythrocytes depends on (i) oxidative injury (formation of methemoglobin, Heinz bodies, membrane injury and RBC destruction), (ii) aging and normal lifespan (metabolic impairment, cumulative oxidative damage and senescent RBC antigens) and (iii) anemia of newborn [14]. Erythrocyte disorders have a direct relationship with various forms of anemia and it is essential to diagnose these disorders at an early stage. An accurate diagnosis would then pave way for specific and appropriate treatment and management strategies for each disorder. Transfusions are generally employed to reduce the severity of erythrocyte disorders. Better blood banking and increased availability of blood would provide far reaching effects into the treatment of erythrocyte disorders.

REFERENCES

[1] Hall, J. E. and Guyton, C. A. 2011. *Guyton and Hall Textbook of Medical Physiology E-Book*. Philadelphia: Elsevier Health Sciences.

[2] Kaushansky, K., Lichtman, M. A., Prchal, J. T., Levi, M., Press, O. W., Burns, L. J. and Caliguiri, M. A. 2016. *Williams Hematology*. New York: McGraw-Hill Education.

[3] Mohandas, N. and Gallagher P. G. 2008. "Red cell membrane: past, present, and future." *Blood* 112: 3939-3948.

[4] Harmening, D. M. 2018. *Modern Blood Banking & Transfusion Practices*. New York: FA Davis.

[5] Xiuli, A. and Mohandas, N. 2008. "Disorders of red cell membrane." *British Journal of Haematology* 141: 367-375.

[6] Prankerd, T. A. J. 1955. "The metabolism of the human erythrocyte: a review." *British Journal of Haematology* 1: 131-145.

[7] Steck, T. L. 1974. "The organization of proteins in the human red blood cell membrane: a review." *The Journal of Cell Biology* 62: 1-19.

[8] Tanner, M. J. A. 1983. "Erythrocyte membrane structure and function." In *Malaria and the Red Cell*, 3-23. London: Pitman.

[9] Petty, H. R. and Richard, C. J. 1994. *Molecular Biology of Membranes: Structure and Function.* New York: Springer Science and Business media.

[10] Mathews, C. K., van Holde, K. E. and Ahern, K. G. 2000. *Biochemistry* (3rd ed.). San Francisco: Addison-Wesley.

[11] Sabban, E., Marchesi, V., Adesnik, M. and Sabatini, D. D. 1981. "Erythrocyte membrane protein band 3: its biosynthesis and incorporation into membranes." *Journal of Cell Biology* 91: 637-646.

[12] Wang, D. N. 1994. "Band 3 protein: structure, flexibility and function." *FEBS Letters* 346: 26-31.

[13] Steck, T. L. 1978 "The band 3 protein of the human red cell membrane: a review." *Journal of Supramolecular Structure* 8: 311-324.

[14] Harvey, J. W. 1997. "The erythrocyte: physiology, metabolism, and biochemical disorders." In *Clinical Biochemistry of Domestic Animals (Fifth Edition)*, 157-203. Cambridge: Academic Press.

[15] Morris, M. B. and Lux, S. E. 1995. "Characterization of the binary interaction between human erythrocyte protein 4.1 and actin." *European Journal of Biochemistry* 231: 644-650.

[16] Gallagher, P. G. 2005. "Red cell membrane disorders." *ASH Education Program Book* 1: 13-18.

[17] Delaunay, J. 2002. "Molecular basis of red cell membrane disorders." *Acta Haematologica* 108: 210-218.

[18] Mohandas, N. and Evan, E. 1994. "Mechanical properties of the red cell membrane in relation to molecular structure and genetic defects." *Annual Review of Biophysics and Biomolecular Structure* 23: 787-818.

[19] Diez-Silva, M., Dao, M., Han, J., Lim, C. and Suresh, S. 2010. "Shape and biomechanical characteristics of human red blood cells in health and disease." *MRS Bulletin* 35: 382-388.

[20] Costa, L., Galimand, J., Fenneteau, O. and Mohandas, N. 2013. "Hereditary spherocytosis, elliptocytosis, and other red cell membrane disorders." *Blood Reviews* 27: 167-178.

[21] Beutler, E. 1975. "Genetic disorders of human red blood cells." *JAMA* 233: 1184-1188.

[22] Pivkin, I. V., Peng, Z., Karniadakis G. E., Buffet, P. A., Dao, M. and Suresh, S. 2016. "Biomechanics of red blood cells in human spleen and

consequences for physiology and disease." *Proceedings of the National Academy of Sciences* 113: 7804-7809.

[23] Dhermy, D., Schrével, J. and Lecomte, M-C. 2007. "Spectrin-based skeleton in red blood cells and malaria." *Current Opinion in Hematology* 14: 198-202.

[24] Tse, W. T. and Lux, S. E. 1999. "Red blood cell membrane disorders." *British Journal of Haematology* 104: 2-13.

[25] Zarkowsky, H. S., Mohandas, N., Speaker C. B. and Shohet, S. B. 1975. "A congenital hemolytic anemia with thermal sensitivity of the erythrocyte membrane." *British Journal of Haematology* 29: 537-543.

[26] Mohandas, N. and Xiuli, A. 2012. "Malaria and human red blood cells." *Medical Microbiology and Immunology* 201: 593-598.

[27] Rosanas-Urgell, A., Lin, E., Manning, L., Rarau, P., Laman, M., Senn, N., Grimberg, B. T., Tavul, L., Stanisic, D. I., Robinson, L. J., Aponte, J. J., Dabod, E., Reeder, J. C., Siba, P., Zimmerman, P. A., Davis, T. M., King, C. L., Michon, P. and Mueller, I. 2012. "Reduced risk of *Plasmodium vivax* malaria in Papua New Guinean children with Southeast Asian ovalocytosis in two cohorts and a case-control study." *PLoS Medicine* 9: e1001305.

[28] Mohandas, N., Winardi, R., Knowles, D., Leung, A., Parra, M., George, E., Conboy, J. and Chasis, J. 1992. "Molecular basis for membrane rigidity of hereditary ovalocytosis. A novel mechanism involving the cytoplasmic domain of band 3." *The Journal of Clinical Investigation* 89: 686-692.

[29] King, M-J. and Zanella, A. 2013. "Hereditary red cell membrane disorders and laboratory diagnostic testing." *International Journal of Laboratory Hematology* 35: 237-243.

[30] Iolascon, A., Perrotta, S. and Stewart, W. 2003. "Red blood cell membrane defects." *Reviews in Clinical and Experimental Hematology* 7: 22-56.

[31] Bruce, L. J., Robinson, H. C., Guizouarn, H., Borgese, F., Harrison, P., King, M. J., Goede, J. S., Coles, S. E., Gore, D. M., Lutz, H. U., Ficarella, R., Layton, D. M., Iolascon, A., Ellory, J. C. and Stewart, G. W. 2005. "Monovalent cation leaks in human red cells caused by single amino-acid substitutions in the transport domain of the band 3 chloride-bicarbonate exchanger, AE1." *Nature Genetics* 37: 1258-1263.

[32] Zarychanski, R., Schulz, V. P., Houston, B. L., Maksimova, Y., Houston, D. S., Smith, B., Rinehart, J. and Gallagher, P. G. 2012. "Mutations in the mechanotransduction protein PIEZO1 are associated with hereditary xerocytosis." *Blood* 120: 1908-1915.

[33] Helen, R. M. and Lehmann, H. 2013. "The Hemoglobinopathies. " In *The Red Blood Cell Vol. 2*. Cambridge: Academic Press.

[34] Rogers, K. 2010. *Blood: Physiology and Circulation*. Chicago: Britannica Educational Publishing.

[35] Kato, G. J., Piel, F. B., Reid, C. D., Gaston, M. H., Ohene-Frempong, K., Krisnamurti, L., Smith, W. R., Panepinto, J. A., Weatherall, D. J., Costa, F. F. and Vichensky, E. P. 2018. "Sickle cell disease." *Nature Reviews Disease Primers* 4: 18010.

[36] Piel, F. B., Steinberg, M. H. and Rees, D. C. 2017. "Sickle cell disease." *New England Journal of Medicine* 376: 1561-1573.

[37] Bain, B. J. 2014. *Blood Cells: A Practical Guide*. New York: John Wiley & Sons.

[38] Rees, D. C., Williams, T. N. and Gladwin, M. T. 2010. "Sickle-cell disease." *The Lancet* 376: 2018-2031.

[39] Serjeant, G. R. 1996. "The role of preventive medicine in sickle cell disease." *Journal of the Royal College of Physicians of London* 30: 37-41.

[40] Piel, F. B., Patil, A. P., Howes, R. E., Nyangiri, O. A., Gething, P. W., Dewi, M., Temperley, W. H., Williams, T. N., Weatherall, D. J. and Hay, S. I. 2013. "Global epidemiology of sickle hemoglobin in neonates: a contemporary geostatistical model-based map and population estimates." *The Lancet* 381: 142-151.

[41] Bank, A. L., Rifkind, R. A. and Marks, P. A. 2013. "The Thalassemia Syndromes". In *The Red Blood Cell. Vol. 2*. Cambridge: Academic Press.

[42] Marks, P. A. and Bank, A. 1971. "Molecular pathology of thalassemia syndromes." *Federation Proceedings* 30: 977-982.

[43] Rinehart, J., Gulcicek, E. E., Joiner, C. H., Lifton. R. P. and Gallagher, P. G. 2010. "Determinants of erythrocyte hydration in current opinion in hematology." *Current Opinion in Hematology* 17: 191-197.

[44] Glogowska, E. and Gallagher, P. G. 2015. "Disorders of erythrocyte volume homeostasis." *International Journal of Laboratory Hematology* 37: 85-91.

[45] Halliwell, B. and Gutteridge, J. M. C. 2015. *Free radicals in biology and medicine*. Oxford: Oxford University Press.

[46] Bogdanova, A. and Lutz, H. U. 2013. "Mechanisms tagging senescent red blood cells for clearance in healthy humans." *Frontiers in Physiology* 4: 387.

[47] Orlov, D. and Karkouti., K. 2015. "The pathophysiology and consequences of red blood cell storage." *Anaesthesia* 70: 29-37.

[48] Moxness, M. S., Brunauer, L. S. and Huestis, W. H. 1996. "Hemoglobin oxidation products extract phospholipids from the membrane of human erythrocytes." *Biochemistry* 35: 7181-7187.

[49] Kanner, J. and Harel, S. 1985. "Initiation of membranal lipid peroxidation by activated metmyoglobin and methemoglobin." *Archives of Biochemistry and Biophysics* 237: 314-321.

[50] Kriebardis, A. G., Antonelou, M. H., Stamoulis, K. E., Economou-Petersen, E., Margaritis, L. H. and Papassideri, I. S. 2007. "Progressive oxidation of cytoskeletal proteins and accumulation of denatured hemoglobin in stored red cells." *Journal of Cellular and Molecular Medicine* 11: 148-155.

[51] Welbourn, E. M., Wilson, M. T., Tusof, A., Metodiev, M. V. and Cooper, C. E. 2017. "The mechanism of formation, structure and physiological relevance of covalent hemoglobin attachment to the erythrocyte membrane." *Free Radical Biology and Medicine* 103: 95-106.

[52] Çimen, M. Y. B. 2008. "Free radical metabolism in human erythrocytes." *Clinica Chimica Acta* 390: 1-11.

[53] Fattman, C. L., Schaefer, L. M. and Oury, T. D. 2003. "Extracellular superoxide dismutase in biology and medicine." *Free Radical Biology and Medicine* 35: 236-256.

[54] Facundo, H. T., Brandt, C. T., Owen, J. S. and Lima, V. L. 2004. "Elevated levels of erythrocyte-conjugated dienes indicate increased lipid peroxidation in schistosomiasis mansoni patients." *Brazilian Journal of Medical and Biological Research* 37: 957-962.

[55] Tinmouth, A. and Chin-Yee, I. 2001. "The clinical consequences of the red cell storage lesion." *Transfusion Medicine Reviews* 15: 91-107.

[56] Pavenski, K., Saidenberg, E., Lavoie, M., Tokessy, M. and Branch, D. R. 2012. "Red blood cell storage lesions and related transfusion issues: a

Canadian Blood Services research and development symposium." *Transfusion Medicine Reviews* 26: 68-84.
[57] Kuypers, F. A. 2007. "Membrane lipid alterations in hemoglobinopathies." *ASH Education Program Book* 1: 68-73.
[58] Shacter, E. 2000. "Quantification and significance of protein oxidation in biological samples." *Drug Metabolism Reviews* 32: 307-326.
[59] Dalle-Donne, I., Rossi, R., Giustarini, D., Milzani, A. and Colombo, R. 2003. "Protein carbonyl groups as biomarkers of oxidative stress." *Clinica Chimica Acta* 329: 23-38.
[60] Berlett, B. S. and Stadtman, E. R. 1997. "Protein oxidation in aging, disease, and oxidative stress." *Journal of Biological Chemistry* 272: 20313-20316.
[61] Thomas, J. A. and Mallis, R. J. 2001. "Aging and oxidation of reactive protein sulfhydryls." *Experimental Gerontology* 36: 1519-1526.
[62] Witko-Sarsat, V., Gausson, V. and Descamps-Latscha, B. 2003. "Are advanced oxidation protein products potential uremic toxins?" *Kidney International* 63: S11-S14.
[63] Adly, A. A. M. 2010. "Oxidative stress and disease: an updated review." *Research Journal of Immunology* 3: 129-145.
[64] Aruoma, O. I. 1998. "Free radicals, oxidative stress, and antioxidants in human health and disease." *Journal of the American Oil Chemists' Society* 75: 199-212.
[65] Schrag, M., Mueller, C., Zabel, M., Crofton, A., Kirsch, W. M., Ghribi, O., Squitti, R. and Perry, G. 2013. "Oxidative stress in blood in Alzheimer's disease and mild cognitive impairment: a meta-analysis." *Neurobiology of Disease* 59: 100-110.
[66] Pohanka, M. 2013. "Role of oxidative stress in infectious diseases. A review." *Folia Microbiologica* 58: 503-513.
[67] Corrons, J-L. V. 2009. "Red blood cell enzyme defects." *ESH Handbook on Disorders of Erythropoiesis, Erythrocytes and Iron Metabolism* 17: 436-453.
[68] Gregg, X. T. and Prchal, J. T. 2005. "Red cell enzymes." *ASH Education Program Book* 1: 19-23.
[69] Beutler, E. 1972. "Disorders due to enzyme defects in the red blood cell." In *Advances in Metabolic Disorders*, 131-160. New York: Elsevier.

[70] van Wijk, R. and van Solinge, W. W. 2005. "The energy-less red blood cell is lost: erythrocyte enzyme abnormalities of glycolysis." *Blood* 106: 4034-4042.

[71] Zanella, A., Bianchi, P. and Fermo, E. 2009. "Red cell enzyme deficiencies: molecular and clinical aspects." In *Hematology Meeting Reports* (formerly *Haematologica Reports*).

[72] Beutler, E. 1979. "Red cell enzyme defects as nondiseases and as diseases." *Blood* 54: 1-7.

[73] Grace, R. F. and Glader, B. 2018. "Red Blood Cell Enzyme Disorders." *Pediatric Clinics of North America* 65: 579-595.

[74] Kugler, W. and Lakomek, M. 2000. "Glucose-6-phosphate isomerase deficiency." *Best Practice & Research Clinical Haematology* 13: 89-101.

[75] Valentine, W. N. 1972. "Red cell enzyme deficiencies as a cause of hemolytic disorders." *Annual Review of Medicine* 23: 93-100.

[76] Fujii, H. and Miwa, S. 2000. "Other erythrocyte enzyme deficiencies associated with non-hematological symptoms: phosphoglycerate kinase and phosphofructokinase deficiency." *Best Practice & Research Clinical Haematology* 13: 141-148.

[77] Beutler, E., Scott, S., Bishop, A., Margolis, N., Matsumoto, F. and Kuhl, W. 1973. "Red cell aldolase deficiency and hemolytic anemia: a new syndrome." *Transactions of the Association of American Physicians* 86: 154.

[78] Beutler, E. 1975. *Red cell metabolism: a manual of biochemical methods*. London: Grune & Stratton.

[79] Daar, I. O., Artymiuk, P. J., Phillips, D. C. and Maquat, L. E. 1986. "Human triose-phosphate isomerase deficiency: a single amino acid substitution results in a thermolabile enzyme." *Proceedings of the National Academy of Sciences* 83: 7903-7907.

[80] Schneider, A., Westwood, B., Yim, C., Prchal, J., Berkow, R., Labotka, R., Warrier, R. and Beutler, E. 1995. "Triosephosphate isomerase deficiency: repetitive occurrence of point mutation in amino acid 104 in multiple apparently unrelated families." *American Journal of Hematology* 50: 263-268.

[81] Noel, N., Flanagan, J., Kalko, S. G., Bajo, M. J. R., Manu, M. M, Fuster, J. L. G., Beutler, E. and Corrons, J-L. V. 2006. "Two new

phosphoglycerate kinase mutations associated with chronic hemolytic anemia and neurological dysfunction in two patients from Spain." *British Journal of Haematology* 132: 523-529.

[82] Michelson, A. M., Blake, C. C., Evans, S. T. and Orkin, S. H. 1985. "Structure of the human phosphoglycerate kinase gene and the intron-mediated evolution and dispersal of the nucleotide-binding domain." *Proceedings of the National Academy of Sciences* 82: 6965-6969.

[83] Rosa, R., Calvin, M. C., Prehu, M. O. and Arous, N. 1984. "Purification of human erythrocyte phosphoglyceromutase." *Journal of Chromatography A* 285: 203-209.

[84] de Atauri, P., Repiso, A., Oliva, B., Corrons, J-L. V., Climent, F. and Carreras, J. 2005. "Characterization of the first described mutation of human red blood cell phosphoglycerate mutase." *Biochimica et Biophysica Acta (BBA)-Molecular Basis of Disease* 1740: 403-410.

[85] Brown, K. A. 2015. "Erythrocyte Metabolism and Enzyme Defects." *Laboratory Medicine* 27: 329-333.

[86] Glader, B. 2009. "Hereditary hemolytic anemias due to red blood cell enzyme disorders." In *Wintrobe's Clinical Hematology.* 12th ed. Philadelphia: Lippincott Williams and Wilkins.

[87] Mahendra, P. 1992. "Pyruvate kinase deficiency: association with G6PD deficiency." *British Medical Journal* 305: 760-763.

[88] Tanaka, K. R. and Paglia, D. E. 1971. "Pyruvate kinase deficiency." *Seminars in Hematology* 8: 367-396.

[89] Beutler, E. and Gelbart, T. 2000. "Estimating the prevalence of pyruvate kinase deficiency from the gene frequency in the general white population." *Blood* 95: 3585-3588.

[90] Steensma, D. P., Hoyer, J. D. and Fairbanks, V. F. 2001. "Hereditary red blood cell disorders in middle eastern patients." In *Mayo Clinic Proceedings* 76: 285-293. London: Elsevier.

[91] Miwa, S., Nishina, T., Kakehashi, Y., Kitamura, M. and Hiratsuka, A. 1971. "Studies on erythrocyte metabolism in a case with hereditary deficiency of H-subunit of lactate dehydrogenase." *Nihon Ketsueki Gakkai Zasshi: Journal of Japan Haematological Society* 34: 228.

[92] Kremer, J. P., Datta, T., Pretsch, W., Charles, D. J. and Dörmer, P. 1987. "Mechanisms of compensation of hemolytic anemia in a lactate dehydrogenase mouse mutant." *Experimental Hematology* 15: 664-670.

[93] Vani, R., Ravikumar, S., Krishnegowda, M. and Hsieh, C. 2015. "Storage lesions in blood components." *Oxidants and Antioxidants in Medical Science* 4: 125-132.
[94] Chiarelli, L. R., Fermo, E., Zanella, A. and Valentini, G. 2006. "Hereditary erythrocyte pyrimidine 5′-nucleotidase deficiency: a biochemical, genetic and clinical overview." *Hematology* 11: 67-72.
[95] Jaffe, E. R. 1995. "Cytochrome b5 reductase deficiency and enzymopenic hereditary methemoglobinemia." In *The metabolic and molecular basis of inherited disease*. New York: McGraw-Hill.
[96] Bain, B. J. 2017. *A beginner's guide to blood cells*. New Jersey: John Wiley & Sons.
[97] Nola, M. and Snjezˇana, D. 2009. The hematopoietic and lymphoid systems. In *Pathology secrets*. New York: Elsevier Health Sciences.

BIOGRAPHICAL SKETCHES

R. Soumya

Affiliation: Department of Biotechnology, JAIN (Deemed-to-be University), Bengaluru, Karnataka, India

Education:
- Ph.D. in Biotechnology, 2018 from JAIN (Deemed-to-be University), Bengaluru.
- Master's degree in Health Science, 2010 from Savitribhai Phule University of Pune, Pune.
- Bachelor's degree [CBZ] 2008 from Mount Carmel College, Bengaluru

Research and Professional Experience: 6 years of Research experience

Honors: Awarded INSPIRE-DST fellowship from 2012 by the government of India.

Publications from the Last 3 Years:

- Carl, H., Soumya, R. and Vani, R. 2018. "Ferric reducing ability of plasma: A potential marker in stored plasma." *Asian Journal of Transfusion Science.* In Press.
- Soumya, R. and Vani, R. 2017. "Vitamin C as a modulator of oxidative stress in erythrocytes of stored blood. *Acta Haematologica Polonica* 48: 350-356.
- Carl. H., Soumya, R., Srinivas, P. and Vani, R. 2016. "Oxidative stress in erythrocytes of banked ABO blood." *Hematology* 21: 630-634.
- Manasa, K., Soumya, R. and Vani, R. 2016. "Phytochemicals as potential therapeutics for thrombocytopenia. *Journal of Thrombosis and Thrombolysis* 41: 436-440.
- Soumya, R., Carl, H. and Vani, R. 2016. "Prospects of curcumin as an additive in storage solutions: a study on erythrocytes." *Turkish Journal of Medical Science* 46: 825-833.
- Soumya, R. and Vani, R. 2016. "Comparison of the protective nature of antioxidants on stored erythrocytes." *Applied Medical Research* doi:10.5455/amr.20160309115846

R. Vani

Affiliation: Department of Biotechnology, JAIN (Deemed-to-be University), Bengaluru, Karnataka, India

Education:
- Ph.D. in Zoology, 2008 from Bangalore University, Bengaluru.
- Master's degree in Zoology, 1997 from Bangalore University.
- Bachelor's degree [CBZ] 1995 from Vijaya College, Bengaluru

Research and Professional Experience: 16 years of Research experience and 12 years of professional experience.

Professional Appointments:
- Associate Professor in Biotechnology, School of Sciences-PG, JAIN (Deemed-to-be University), Bangalore from July 2018 till date. (Courses: Molecular Genetics, Cell Biology, Molecular Biology, Genetic Engineering and Animal Biotechnology).
- Assistant Professor in Biotechnology, School of Sciences-PG, JAIN (Deemed-to-be University), Bangalore from 21st May 2008 till June 2018. (Courses: Molecular Genetics, Cell Biology, Molecular Biology, Genetic Engineering and Animal Biotechnology).
- Lecturer in Biology, VET College, Bangalore for two years from July 2000 to June 2002.

Honors:
- Awarded VGST-SMYSR funding for Seed Money to Young Scientists for Research, in 2013, from the government of Karnataka.
- Qualified the CSIR [NET] JRF test in 2002, ranked one among the top 100 and eligible for Shyam Prasad Mukherjee Fellowship Exam.

Publications from the Last 3 Years:
- Manasa, K. and Vani, R. 2018 "L-carnitine as an additive in Tyrode's buffer during platelet storage." *Blood Coagulation and Fibrinolysis* 29:613-621.
- Manasa, K. and Vani, R. 2018. "Platelet storage: Role of *Cassia tora* Linn." *Asian Journal of Transfusion Science* In Press.
- Carl, H., Soumya, R, and Vani, R. "Ferric reducing ability of plasma: A potential marker in stored plasma." *Asian Journal of Transfusion Science* In Press
- Soumya, R. and Vani, R. 2017. "Vitamin C as a modulator of oxidative stress in erythrocytes of stored blood." *Acta Haematologica Polonica* 48: 350-356.
- Carl, H. and Vani, R. 2017. "Influence of L-carnitine on stored rat blood: A study on plasma. *Turkish Journal of Hematology* 34: 328-333.
- Carl, H., Soumya, R., Srinivas, P. and Vani, R. 2016. "Oxidative stress in erythrocytes of banked ABO blood." *Hematology* 21: 630-634.

- Manasa, K., Soumya, R. and Vani, R. 2016. "Phytochemicals as potential therapeutics for thrombocytopenia. *Journal of Thrombosis and Thrombolysis*. 41: 436-440.
- Soumya, R., Carl, H. and Vani, R. 2016. "Prospects of curcumin as an additive in storage solutions: a study on erythrocytes." *Turkish Journal of Medical Science* 46: 825-833.
- Manasa, K. and Vani, R. 2016. "Influence of oxidative stress on stored platelets," *Advances in. Hematolology* doi:10.1155/2016/4091461.
- Soumya, R. and Vani, R. 2016. "Comparison of the protective nature of antioxidants on stored erythrocytes." *Applied Medical Research* doi:10.5455/amr.20160309115846.

In: Erythrocytes
Editor: Katy Jorissen

ISBN: 978-1-53615-914-1
© 2019 Nova Science Publishers, Inc.

Chapter 3

ERYTHROCYTE MEMBRANES: UNIQUE CONSTITUENT OF BIOLOGICAL/HYBRID DRUG DELIVERY SYSTEMS

Ivana T. Drvenica[1],*, PhD, Ana Z. Stančić[1],
Branko M. Bugarski[2], PhD, Ivana Pajic-Lijaković[2], PhD,
Irina Maslovarić[1], PhD and Vesna Lj. Ilić[1], PhD

[1]Institute for Medical Research, University of Belgrade,
Belgrade, Serbia
[2]Faculty of Technology and Metallurgy, University of Belgrade,
Belgrade, Serbia

ABSTRACT

For many decades, the red blood cell membranes were in focus of research interest solely as a model system for investigation into the various membrane-related phenomena, composition/organization or membrane transport properties, as well as the comparative proteomic and lipidomic analyses in health and disease. During 50s, along with the first

---

* Corresponding Author's E-mail: ivana.drvenica@imi.bg.ac.rs.

experimental steps in ATP encapsulation in erythrocytes membranes, these entities begin to fascinate clinicians and researchers by their super carrier capabilities for the controlled and targeted delivery (vascular, pulmonary, subcutaneous) of wide range of conventional drugs and biologicals. A relatively new realm for erythrocyte membrane is its application in targeted delivery of nanoparticles, like erythrocyte membrane cloaked nanoparticles, incorporating their most useful traits such as long circulation and stealth features.

This chapter focuses on red blood cell membrane as unique constituent of drug delivery systems, including nano-sized ones (nanoerythrosomes) and *ex vivo* technologies for their preparation. Rheological characterization of membranes as well as the change induced by various experimental conditions is prerequisite for their application as drug carriers. The membrane viscoelasticity described by appropriate constitutive model is related to kinetic of drug release in order to whole process optimization. Furthermore, chapter will bring review of developed hybrid drug delivery vehicles of erythrocyte membranes as natural bio-derivative material, and nanoparticles, mainly made of synthetic material, whose combined advantages serve as immunologically non-invasive drug delivery platform. The advantages and drawbacks are specifically summarized to get critical point of view on existing and future medical applications of erythrocyte membrane as drug carriers. As an example of complexity in research toward development of such erythrocyte membrane based drug delivery systems starting from animal erythrocyte, morphological, biochemical and drug release profile assessment will be reviewed.

Keywords: red blood cells, erythrocyte membrane, erythrocyte ghosts, drug delivery systems, encapsulation

1. INTRODUCTION

Nowadays, drug delivery system is entering a quite challenging era. The uncertainty of the outcome of billions of euros worth projects on the development of new drug molecules discourage even the richest countries from researching and the development of new drug entities. That is the reason why modern pharmacotherapy is more and more turning to the improvement of the effects of already existing active substances through the development of new pharmaceutical forms, sophisticated drug carriers or so called drug delivery systems (DDS). Current research in drug delivery aimes to maximize the therapeutic efficacy of drugs and minimize the adverse effects, by means of prolonged, targeted and site-specific DDS (Jain and Jain 2003). Thus, modern DDS cover systems that represent simple, soluble macromolecules (such as monoclonal antibodies, soluble synthetic polymers, polysaccharides and biodegradable polymers), but also a much more complex multicomponent particle structures (microcapsules, microparticles, liposomes, lipoproteins, cells and cellular membrane (ghosts)). Progressively more, cell-based delivery systems have an advantage over available natural or synthetic carriers (Yoo et al. 2011) since they can meet clinical expectations in treatment of many "modern age" diseases. For this reason, increasing attention of researchers and clinicians is attracted to biological carriers derived from bacterial and mammalian cells (Lautenschläger et al. 2014). Different kinds of cells have been used as novel drug delivery systems, including erythrocytes, platelets, leukocytes, stem cells, fibroblasts, hepatocytes and cancer cells (Hamidi et al. 2007a). Among them, the erythrocytes have been the most investigated and it is found that they possess huge clinical potential in controlled/prolonged/targeted delivery of drugs (Muzykantov 2010; Villa et al. 2017; Millán, Bravo and Lanao 2017; Han, Wang and Liu 2018). This is supported by the fact that the systems of autologous human erythrocytes loaded with L-aspariganase and dexamethasone sodium phosphate have been under the clinical trials (Phase 1 and 3, respectively (www.clinicaltrial.gov) during the past two decades. These procedures, from the pharmacokinetic and pharmacodynamic aspects, have provided very satisfactory results in the treatment of severe inflammatory/malignant diseases without associated side effects (Rossi et al. 2004; Bossa et al. 2013; Villa et al. 2016; 2017).

Generally, erythrocytes participate in the distribution and metabolism of more than 50 biologically active substances (e.g., captopril, haloperidol, heroin, testosterone, insulin, catecholamines, penicillamine, daunorubicin) (Hinderling 1997). Erythrocytes thus, "unintentionally" serve as natural blood compartments that participate in the pharmacokinetics, biodistribution, metabolism, release, and the mechanism of action of various drugs. However, the intentional use of erythrocytes and their membranes as a carrier for the delivery of biologically active substances is of much greater interest. In the early seventies of the twentieth century it was assumed that the effects of certain drugs could be improved by their encapsulation in autologous or immunologically compatible donor erythrocytes. This way enables relatively precise, controlled and prolonged release of encapsulated drug substance (Ihler, Glew and Schnure 1973). The newest proposed strategies for fabrication of erythrocyte-based delivery systems include even genetic engineering approaches (Han, Wang and Liu 2018). It is known that mature erythrocytes do not contain any genetic materials, which minimizes the safety risks compared to other gene and cell therapies (Luk and Zhang 2015), but limits their genetically modification (Han, Wang and Liu 2018). Recently erythroid precursors (hematopoietic stem cells) are engineered with the aim to express specific proteins on mature erythrocytes, which make them acting as therapeutics (Shi et al. 2014; Huang et al. 2017; Pishesha et al. 2017).

In order to emphasize the huge potential of intrinsic properties of erythrocyte membrane, which enables the use of erythrocytes as DDS (without performing genetic engineering modification), we should refer to the first studies on encapsulation of organic compounds of metabolic interest in erythrocyte ghosts in concentrations higher than those found in the original intact cells (Gardos 1953, Gourley 1957). These studies revealed remarkable trait of erythrocyte membrane integrity, meaning that it can be restored/resealed in isotonic saline, after lysis in hypotonic buffer. If most of the hemoglobin leaked out, the resealed cell appears pale which is known as 'ghost'. If most of the hemoglobin and other cellular constituents are retained, the cell preserves most of the properties of normal erythrocytes and probably should be referred as a resealed erythrocyte (Ihler 1983). However, the resulting erythrocyte ghost characteristics are method- and species- dependent and should be specified in each of the cases reported (Hoffman 1992; Kostić et al. 2014); this will be further discussed in detail (see section 2 and 6). Over the decades researchers realized that erythrocytes are carriers "designed by Mother Nature" (Muzykantov 2010), allowing many other *ex-vivo/in-vivo* manipulation methods besides encapsulation, such absorption and bioconjugation to the erythrocyte surface to finely control drug delivery (Han, Wang and Liu 2018). Thus, the strategies in erythrocyte/erythrocyte membrane use (Figure 1) so far include: encapsulation of biologically active compounds into erythrocytes (a) and "empty" erythrocyte membranes (b), bounding of biologically active compounds to the surface of erythrocytes (c), binding of nanoparticles with encapsulated drug to the surface of erythrocyte membranes (d), binding of conjugated drug by specific molecules on the surface of erythrocyte membranes *in vivo* (e), use of erythrocyte membrane with encapsulated drug as nuclei for microcapsule formation (f), extrusion of erythrocyte membranes encapsulating drug to obtain nanoerythrosomes (g) and nano-sized erythrocyte membranes enveloping nanoparticles (h).

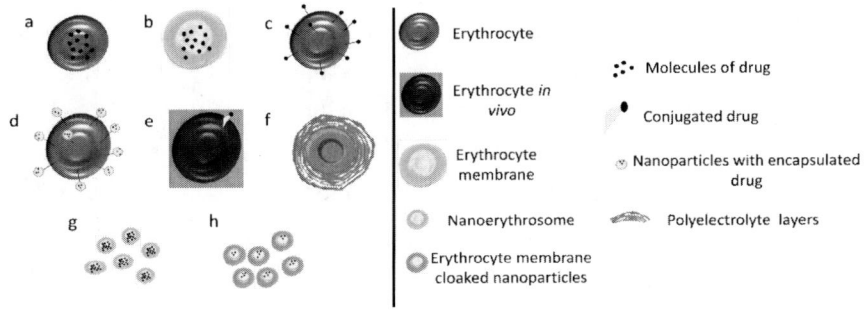

Figure 1. Different approaches in use of erythrocytes and erythrocyte membranes as drug delivery systems.

Encapsulation of active compounds in erythrocytes/erythrocyte membranes is the oldest method related to the erythrocyte use as DDS; however, it remains the most employed method to date (Figure 1a and 1b). This methodology is limited to the drugs that have high solubility in water, as well as metabolic stability against erythrocyte enzymes if the intact erythrocytes are used (Yousefpour and Chilkoti 2014). On the other hand, the presence of those hydrolytic enzymes in the interior space of erythrocytes can be used as a strategy for bioconversion of pro- drugs, i.e., use of erythrocytes as long circulating drug bioreactors (Biagiotti et al. 2011). The aforementioned approach (Figure 1a) also includes encapsulation of additional drug loaded carrier into erythrocytes, as it was demonstrated in the case of chitosan particles containing drug sodium valproate encapsulated into human erythrocytes (Hamidi et al. 2011).

Other experimental approaches in application of erythrocytes for intravascular drug delivery is the conjugation of pharmacologically active compounds onto the surface of erythrocytes through molecules expressed on their surface (Figure 1c). For instance, erythrocytes were used as delivery carriers for thrombolytic agents including tissue-type plasminogen activators (tPAs) and recombinant soluble urokinase plasminogen activator receptors (Yoo et al. 2011). Molecules of tPA coupled to the surface of erythrocytes persisted in bloodstream at least tenfold longer than the free tPA (Murciano et al. 2003), allowing conversion of tPA into thromboprophylactic agent as a useful step of novel approach for preventing cerebrovascular thrombosis (Danielyan et al. 2008).

Further methods in the development of erythrocyte based drug delivery systems include the polymeric nanoparticles anchoring to the surface of erythrocytes (Figure 1d) in order to prolong their vascular half-life and robustness (Chambers and Mitragotri 2004); as proposed by the same authors this strategy is effective for nanoparticles ranging in diameter from 100 nm to 1.1 µm. This cellular hitchhiking strategy can solve major issues in nanoparticle-based therapeutic strategies: the avoidance of metabolic organs such as liver and spleen and the accumulation of nanoparticles to sites that is difficult to reach such as lungs and brain (Brenner et al. 2018; Han, Wang and Liu 2018). Besides, other approaches in application of erythrocytes as drug carriers involve *in vivo* binding of active compounds to erythrocytes by molecules that have specific affinity for erythrocytes (Figure 1e). For instance, Zaitsev and co-workers managed to conjugate tPA to a monoclonal antibody against complement receptor type 1 primarily expressed on human erythrocytes (Zaitsev et al. 2006). Screening a naive phage-displayed library against the whole mouse erythrocytes yielded a 12 amino acid peptide that binds to the surface of erythrocyte with high specificity and has been introduced as new strategy for improving pharmacokinetic profile of proteins used for therapeutic purpose (Kontos and Hubbell 2010). This approach of using drug conjugated to erythrocytes *in vivo* avoids the erythrocytes isolation procedure and *ex vivo* manipulation, thus eliminating the risk of contamination, but raises the cost by stepping into the field of personalized medicine.

Bioengineering based methods have shown successful application of erythrocyte membrane (ghosts) as nuclei (Figure 1f) for formulation of multilayer polyelectrolyte microcapsules (*Layer by layer*, LbL), which can be used for controlled and prolonged release of substance encapsulated in erythrocyte ghosts (Georgieva et al. 2004; Kreft et al. 2006; Shaillender et al. 2011). Nanoerythrosomes are one more DDS entity prepared by the extrusion of erythrocyte ghosts, with the average diameter of 100 nm (Zhang 2016). Diagnocure Inc., Canada, patented polyethyleneglycol conjugated nanoerythrosomes as erythrocyte ghosts nano-vesicles having a decreased immunogenic potential for use in diagnostic and therapeutic purposes ("EP0929317A2, Google Patents" 2019). For instance, it was shown that daunorubicin covalently linked to nanoerythrosomes has the cytotoxicity as high as the free daunorubicin, but higher antineoplastic activity than that of the free drug (Lejeune et al. 1994; Moorani et al. 1996). These first studies on nanoerythrosomes open a new research realm toward use of erythrocyte membranes as "camouflaging" cover of synthetic nanoparticles to act as biomimetic delivery platform. The hybrid DDS made of erythrocyte membranes provide the opportunity to actively inhibit the clearance of their therapeutic load by immune system, thereby improving drug pharmacokinetics and pharmacodynamics (Luk 2016). For instance, biomimetic properties of autologous erythrocyte membranes were used to coat biodegradable polymeric poly(lactic-co-glycolic acid) (PLGA) nanoparticles, thus successfully by-passing macrophage uptake and systemic clearance of these particles (Figure 1h) (Hu et al. 2011).

In this chapter, special attention will be provided to fundamental properties of mammalian erythrocyte membrane that can be used to develop new carriers for drugs and diagnostic agents. There are excellent recent reviews and studies on the strategy outlining the ideology, methodology and outcomes of animal and human studies on coupling of active agents onto the surface of erythrocytes *ex vivo/in vivo* and use of intact erythrocytes as drug carriers/bioreactors (Rossi et al. 2016; Villa et al. 2017; Han, Wang and Liu 2018; Brenner et al. 2018), but they will not be discussed in this chapter. It would be impossible to delineate all aspects of erythrocyte based drug delivery strategies in a reasonably concise chapter. Instead, we will mainly focus on application of erythrocyte membranes as constituents of DDS, when their unique intrinsic properties allow their application as drug vehicles and determine the overall features of prepared DDS, like in strategies presented in Figure 1b, h, g.

2. Biological Traits of Erythrocyte/ Erythrocyte Membrane Determine Their Advantages/Disadvantages as Constituents of DDS

Erythrocytes or red blood cells are the most common cellular components of the blood (>99%) of all vertebrates. One microliter of human blood contains 5 million erythrocytes, i.e., human body has about 30 trillion of erythrocytes. The life span of human erythrocytes lasts 100-120 days. During this period red blood cells, which are anucleate cells, travel ~ 250 km through the cardiovascular system and function as natural oxygen carriers owing to the hemoglobin molecules present in cytosol. Human erythrocytes have a volume of approximately 95 µm and membrane area of ~130 µm, with a diameter of 5 to 7 µm and ~2 µm of thickness. Thus, if used as drug carriers even when they are not completely intact due to inevitable modification by encapsulation procedure (see section 3 and 6), erythrocyte life-span markedly exceed those of other drug delivery systems (e.g., <10 h for PEG-modified "stealth" liposomes) (Muzycantov 2010). The discoid shape of intact erythrocytes gives maximum of elasticity and flexibility, allowing them to pass through very narrow capillary spaces without rupture of the cell membrane. However, fabrication of erythrocyte membrane based DDS, as well as the procedure used for starting erythrocytes manipulation more or less impact the final shape and morphology of these DDS (Kostić et al. 2013; 2014; 2015). Normally, erythrocytes are not subjected to extravasation from circulation to tissues, except in hepatic sinuses and interstitium in the follicles of the spleen, or openings to circulation at the sites of erythrocyte formation and elimination, which are part of the reticuloendothelial system. Macrophages of the reticuloendothelial system in the spleen and liver rapidly and efficiently phagocyte old or membrane damaged or modified erythrocytes. If the erythrocyte based DDS is intended for long intravascular application, this fact can be considered as disadvantageous. On the other hand, this is exactly a natural, direct and effective route for specific intracellular drug targeting by non-intact erythrocyte membrane based delivery system (Sternberg et al. 2011; Fan et al. 2012; Kostić et al. 2014), provided that it is not destroyed by complement in the circulation (Myzikantov 2010). This intentional erythrocyte membrane damage can be also achieved by controlled artificial alteration using Zn dependent cluster rearrangement of the major erythrocyte trans-membrane protein, band 3 (see section 3) (Magnani et al. 1992).

In all cells, including erythrocytes the plasma membrane has several essential functions. These include transport of nutrients into and metabolic wastes out of the cell; preventing unwanted materials in the extracellular milieu from entering the cell and loss of essential metabolites and maintenance of the proper ionic composition, pH ($\approx$7.2), and osmotic pressure of the erythrocyte cytosol (Lodish et al. 2000). To carry out these functions, the erythrocyte membrane contains specific transport proteins that permit the passage of certain small molecules but not others; several of these proteins, use the energy released by ATP hydrolysis to pump ions and other molecules into or out of the cell against their concentration gradients (Lodish et al. 2000). The human erythrocyte membrane consists of 40% lipids (phospholipids, cholesterol, and glycolipids), 50% proteins and 10% carbohydrates. In membranes from human erythrocytes, almost all the sphingomyelin and phosphatidylcholine, both of which have a positively charged head group (see Figure 2), are found in the exoplasmic leaflet. In contrast, lipids with neutral or negative polar head groups (e.g., phosphatidylethanolamine, phosphatidylserine, and phosphatidylinositol) are preferentially located in the cytosolic leaflet (Lodish et al. 2000). Below the membrane there is a cytoskeleton built from the filament of protein spectrin, forming the spectrin network which maintaining the biconcave shape erythrocyte and strengthens the lipid bilayer (Figure 2). The red blood cell membrane skeleton structure represent a pseudohexagonal meshwork of spectrin, actin, protein 4.1R, ankyrin, and actin associated proteins that laminates the inner membrane surface and attaches to the overlying lipid bilayer via band 3–containing multiprotein complexes at the ankyrin- and actin-binding ends of spectrin (Lux 2016). Spectrin α- and β-chains, proteins 4.1, or 4.1R, and actin are the main components of cytoskeleton. These components are connected to each other via two multiprotein complexes: ankyrin and protein 4.1/actin junctional complex. The ankyrin complexes is composed of band 3 tetramers, Rh, RhAG, CD47, glycophorin A and protein 4.2, and the protein 4.1/Actin junctional complex is composed by band 3 dimers binding adducins α- and β-, glycophorin C, GLUT1 and stomatin (Andolfo et al. 2016). Dynamic regulation and cytoskeletal adaptation maintain morphological stability, plasticity and deformability of erythrocytes that are allowing millions of repeated passage through narrow capillaries.

Band 3 is the major red cell membrane protein, with 1.2 million copies per cell (Lux 2016). The molecular mass of band 3 is estimated at approximately 100 kDa. By mild proteolysis, the band 3 protein, which consists of 911 amino acid residues, can be divided into a hydrophilic cytoplasmic fragment of 41 kDa and a hydrophobic membrane fragment of 52 kDa (Aoki 2017). The elongated part of the N-terminal domain facing the cytosol consists of a hydrophilic domain whose ends connect to the hydrophobic domain, and this unit crosses the membrane several times. N terminal part of band 3 is a key attachment site for the membrane skeleton, glycolytic enzymes, and deoxyhemoglobin, where its C-terminal domain forms the red cell anion-exchange channel and aids carbon dioxide transport (Lux 2016; Aoki 2017). Approximately 40% of the band 3 molecules are tetramers in a complex with ankyrin and other integral proteins near the spectrin self-association site (in ankyrin complex). An approximately similar fraction of the band 3 molecules, probably dimers, are located near the spectrin-actin junction and bind to spectrin via protein 4.1R (4.1), protein 4.2 (4.2), and adducin (in actin junctional complex). The remaining band 3 dimers float untethered within the lipid bilayer (unbound band 3) (Lux 2016). Besides its essential structural and metabolic functions, band 3 is the main of all proteins that participate in removal of aged or damaged erythrocytes. In normal undamaged red blood cells band 3 is not aggregated and only a few molecules of naturally-occurring anti-band 3 IgG are bound. In senescent or (oxidative) damaged red blood cells, an aggregation of band 3 occurs, followed by binding of anti-band 3 IgG and complement fragment C3b. Such opsonized erythrocytes are now recognized and eliminated by binding to CR1 or Fc receptors on phagocytes of mononuclear phagocyte system (reticuloendothelial system) (Arese, Turrini and Schwarzer 2005). Besides its importance in removing aged erythrocytes, redistribution of band 3 is of crucial significance in osmotic hemolysis, and all process of drug encapsulation based on osmotic hemolysis. Sato et al. (1993) showed that during rapid hemolysis in hypotonic medium a single large hole opens in the erythrocyte membrane, as a results of swelling of erythrocytes, which is followed by clustering of band 3 (mediated by their cytoplasmic domains) and releasing of hemoglobin. After releasing of hemoglobin, the membrane sealing is accompanied by band 3 redistribution (Sato et al. 1993).

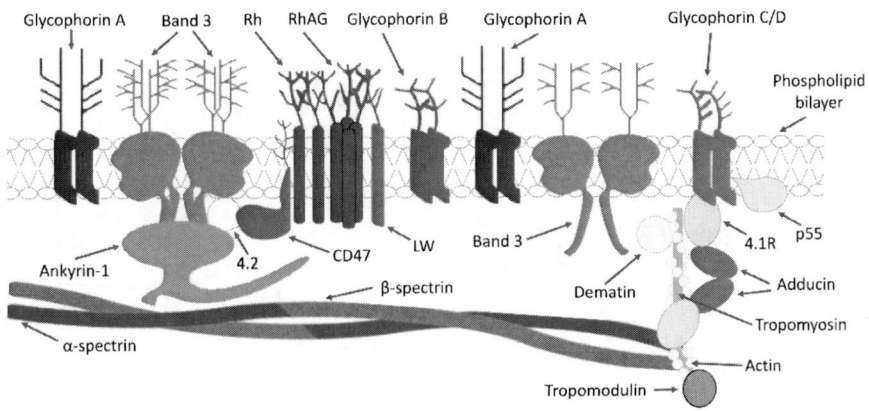

Figure 2. Schematic presentation of the erythrocyte membrane structure. A model of phospholipid bilayer and the major proteins of the erythrocyte membrane are shown: α and β spectrin, ankyrin, band 3 (the anion exchanger), 4.1 (protein 4.1) and 4.2 (protein 4.2), actin, and glycophorin.

Important fact is that the plasma membrane of human erythrocytes in comparison to membranes of other cells can be isolated in near purity, because these cells contain no internal membranes (Lodish et al. 2000). Described human erythrocyte membrane's relative simplicity and ease of isolation has made it the most extensively studied and best understood biological membrane (Jain and Jain 2003). However, if used as drug carriers, due to biological origin, even within the same sample of human blood, erythrocytes can show some inherent variations and be less standardized comparing to other drug delivery systems. These variations include: difference in size, hemoglobin content, levels of oxidative damage, osmotic and mechanic fragility (Sternberg et al. 2011). It is worth noting that each of the mentioned parameters can contribute to their *in vitro/in vivo* performance as drug carriers. Hence, *in vitro* characterization is an important part of studies related to these cellular carriers (Gothoskar 2004). At least it should include osmotic fragility analysis, hemoglobin content, sterility test, shape and surface morphology examined by different microscopy methods (e.g., transmission and scanning electron microscopy, phase contrast microscopy), size distribution and surface potential determined by dynamic light scattering method, and drug content and drug release profile test (via diffusion cell or dialysis method).

What makes these DDS even more complex for studying is that researchers have used various types of mammalian erythrocytes, including erythrocytes of mice, rats, cattle, pigs, dogs, sheep, goats, monkeys, chicken, rabbits (Gothoskar 2004). Investigations on use of membranes originating from erythrocytes of species other than human require additional considerations regarding species- related erythrocytes' properties. These include different life span, size, volume and shape, lipid membrane composition, composition and structural organization of transmembrane and cytoskeletal proteins, enzyme activity, ionic composition, ATP and other metabolites (Jain 1993; Harvey 2008; Pierigè et al. 2017). For instance, erythrocyte survival varies in different animal species from days to months: in small animals, life span of erythrocytes is shorter than those of large ones, and apparently increases with their weights; for instance 55-58 days for murine and rabbit erythrocytes up to

100 days for canine erythrocytes (Pierigè et al. 2017). In order to isolate red blood cells, blood taken by venipuncture is collected and stored for less than two days in heparinized tubes or tubes containing sodium citrate, depending on used specific species blood sample (Gothoskar 2004; Kostić et al. 2013). In research protocols, the erythrocytes are harvested and washed by centrifugation then resuspended in buffer solutions at desired hematocrit values, and stored at 4°C for as long as two days, before their use for drug carrier preparation (Gothoskar 2004; Kostić et al. 2013; Kostić 2015). Another important difference between the human and animal erythrocytes (such as rabbits and cats) often used in preclinical investigations, is the absence of programmed cell death of old/damaged erythrocytes in these animals (Pierigè et al. 2017). Namely, if the prolonged circulation of DDS prepared of erythrocytes from mentioned species is expected, it could vary from the expected life span, since random destruction of erythrocytes is predominant in these animals (Pierigè et al. 2017). Regardless of the method used for encapsulation of active substances within erythrocyte/erythrocyte membranes (see section 3), crucial steps for all procedures are: 1) opening of pores on erythrocyte membrane, which allow entrapping of drug and 2) resealing the pores of the resultant cellular carriers, which allow retention of the entrapped drug. These particular features of erythrocytes that can entrap active substance and still maintain their physiological properties make them almost ideal delivery systems (Villa et al. 2016; Rossi et al. 2016). Erythrocytes that originate from different species show different osmotic properties, therefore the optimal procedure condition of osmosis based methods for erythrocyte pore opening is prerequisite for each species analysis (Kostić et al. 2015). For instance, the recommended osmolality of hypo-osmotic buffers range from 100 mosM/kg in dog erythrocytes, 120 mosM/kg in human erythrocytes, to 200–220 mosM/kg in sheep red blood cells (Millán et al. 2004a). Also, in animals like rats, hemoglobin has very low solubility and it undergoes rapid crystallization (Brunori et al. 1982); this is considered disadvantage because hemoglobin retention is desirable in the process of resealed erythrocyte engineering for drug delivery (Pierigè et al. 2017). A particular issue in designing process for drug encapsulation in

animal erythrocytes is to keep the ability of the membrane to be resealed, since resealing represent a complex phenomenon that requires energy, controlled ionic strength and temperature (Hoffman 1992). This step has to be optimized for erythrocytes of each species in order to achieve the highest encapsulation efficacy (see section 6). Nevertheless, it has been shown that horse, pig, and mouse erythrocytes are about equal in encapsulation potential, while canine red blood cells possess higher encapsulation potential (Pierigè et al. 2017; DeLoach 1985).

As a DDS of biological origin, storage of loaded erythrocyte membranes is an additional limiting factor for their wide-spread clinical use. Therefore, the use of isotonic storage buffers containing essential nutrients (Mg^{2+} and Ca^{2+} ions from $MgCl_2$ and $CaCl_2$, ATP, glucose...), nucleoside or chelators, low temperature storage, liophylization with glycerol or immobilization in alginate gel (Gothoskar 2004) is suggested. Due to the origin of the blood, biological contamination is possible in each step of encapsulation process. Therefore, when working with erythrocyte carriers, rigorous controls are required for their collection and handling (Villa, Seghatchian and Muzykantov 2016).

Since this chapter focuses on methodology of development of erythrocyte membrane based DDS, the next section will summarize the most widely used methods that induce reversible and transient changes in erythrocyte membrane permeability and consequent drug encapsulation. Further, we will discuss modeling approaches of complex phase transition phenomena from erythrocyte to erythrocyte ghost membrane preparations, which occurs in the course of drug encapsulation process into the erythrocyte membranes.

3. METHODS FOR DRUG ENCAPSULATION WITHIN ERYTHROCYTE MEMBRANES

In general, there are three types of methods used for encapsulating active compounds into the erythrocyte membranes: physical, chemical and biological techniques (Figure 3). Physical methods, the most used encapsulation methods, are based on osmosis (Millán et al. 2004b) or electroporation process (Lizano, Pérez and Pinilla 2001). Encapsulation using chemical method is based on perturbation of the membrane, membrane internalization or swelling allowing drug entrapment, after treatment with chemicals such chlorpromazine (Favretto et al. 2013). Biological methods involve some of the known biological phenomena (endocytosis, lipid fusion) in order to accomplish encapsulation of active compound into erythrocytes. For instance, phosphatidylserine-enriched drug loaded liposomes can fuse with the erythrocyte membrane and release the drug content within them (Holovati, Gyongyossy-Issa and Acker 2009; Favretto et al. 2013).

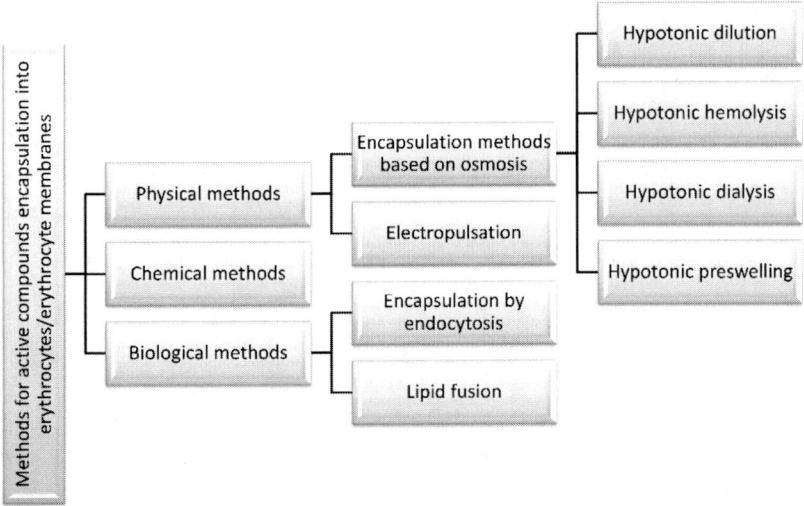

Figure 3. Schematic presentation of methods used for encapsulation of biologically active compounds in erythrocytes and erythrocyte membranes.

Since osmosis based methods appeared to be the most applicable in production of erythrocyte based DDS (Bukara et al. 2016; Ge et al. 2017), general recommendation for successful encapsulation of drugs by this approach include the following: drugs have to be water soluble, resistant to break-down within the erythrocyte membrane, incapable of physical or chemical interactions with erythrocyte membrane and to have well-defined pharmacokinetic and pharmacodynamic characteristics (Hamidi and Tajerzadeh 2003). Several variants of osmosis based procedures for drug encapsulation within the erythrocyte membrane will be in brief summarized in the next section.

3.1. Osmosis Based Methods of Active Substances Encapsulation within Erythrocyte Membranes

3.1.1. Hypotonic Hemolysis

Hypotonic hemolysis method is based on the phenomenon that erythrocytes undergo reversible swelling in hypotonic solution. Under reduced osmotic pressure conditions, erythrocytes swell, and their shape changes from biconcave disks to spheres and the volume of the cells raises (25 – 50%) as the surface remains constant (Millán et al. 2004a; Magnani et al. 1998). Human erythrocytes can compensate osmotic pressure difference between intracellular and extracellular environment to some extent. When the osmolality of surrounding solution exceeds 150 mosM/kg erythrocyte membrane breaks down and the entire cellular content is released. Before the cell lysis, transitory hemolytic openings appear on erythrocyte membrane (diameter 20 – 50 nm) (Fan et al. 2012) and the main intracellular component-hemoglobin leaks through them. Empty erythrocyte membranes or "ghosts" remain after the completed hemolysis process (Hamidi and Tajerzadeh 2003; DeLoach et al. 1980; Stojanović et al. 2012; Pravilovic et al. 2012). If the ghosts are back to the isotonic/hypertonic solution, membrane pores can be closed and original biconcave disk shape is reestablished to some extent. The main disadvantage of hypotonic hemolysis is the lack of the process control, due to the fast exposure of erythrocytes to hypotonic buffer solution, an inevitable rupture of erythrocyte membrane and formation of small vesicles (Figure 4). Vesicles originating from erythrocyte membranes can have structural organization of lipid bilayer opposite to the starting erythrocyte, representing so called "inside-out" vesicles. This could be overcome by gradual introduction of hypotonic buffer into the erythrocyte suspension (Danon 1961; Bugarski and Dovezenski 2000; Stojanović et al. 2012; Kostić et al. 2014; Bukara et al. 2016, Drvenica et al. 2016).

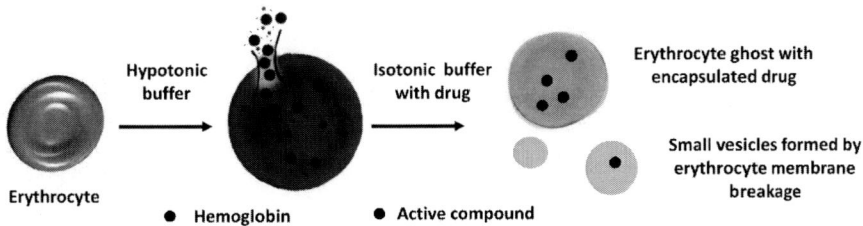

Figure 4. Schematic illustration of hypotonic hemolysis procedure (adapted according to Kostić 2015).

3.1.2. Hypotonic Dilution

Hypotonic dilution was the first method investigated for the encapsulation of chemical compounds into erythrocytes (Figure 5) and it remains the simplest and the fastest one to date (Ihler, Glew and Schnure 1973). In this method, a suspension of packed erythrocytes is diluted with 2-20 times higher volume of aqueous solution of active compound. After the active compound entrapment, the tonicity of suspension is restored by addition of hypertonic buffer. Suspension is then centrifuged, the supernatant is discarded and the pellet is washed with isotonic buffer solution. Using this method, it is possible to obtain so called "white ghosts" (Hamidi and Tajerzadeh 2003). Hypotonic dilution methods used for enzyme encapsulation including beta-glucosidase and beta-galactosidase (Ihler, Glew and Schnure 1973), asparaginase (Deloach and Ihler 1977), bronchodilator drug salbutamol (Bhaskaran and Dhir 1995), as well as anti-inflammatory drug dexamethasone (Rossi et al. 2004) and cholesterol-lowering drug pravastatin (Harisa, Ibrahim and Alanazi 2012) are reported. The main drawback of this procedure is the low entrapment efficiency (Deloach and Ihler, 1977).

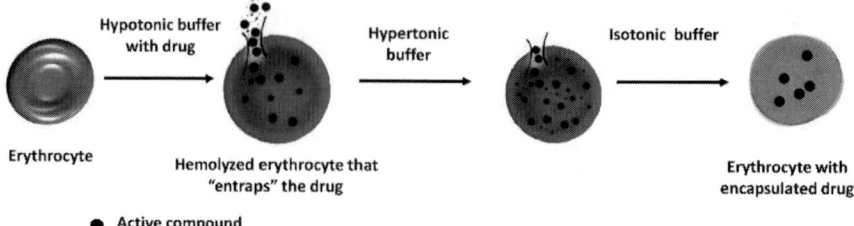

Figure 5. Schematic illustration of hypotonic dilution procedure (adapted according to Kostić 2015).

3.1.3. Hypotonic Pre-Swelling

This method is based on the initial controlled erythrocyte swelling in hypotonic buffer solution (Hamidi and Tajerzadeh 2003). After low speed centrifugation, supernatant is discarded and cell fraction is brought to the lysis point by addition of small amount of aqueous solution of the compound of interest for encapsulation. The tonicity of the cell mixture is restored by adding the hypertonic buffer. Cell suspension is then incubated at 37°C to reseal the hemolytic openings on the erythrocytes (Figure 6). This method is simpler, faster and induces minimal cell destruction in comparison to other encapsulation methods (Jain and Jain 1997). Although different entrapment efficiency is reported, active substance encapsulation using this method include: insulin (Bird, Best and Lewis 1983), primaquine (Talwar and Jaind 1992), enalaprilat (Tajerzadeh and Hamidi 2000), bovine serum albumin (Hamidi et al. 2007b), and pravastatine in form of chitosan nanogel (Harisa et al. 2016).

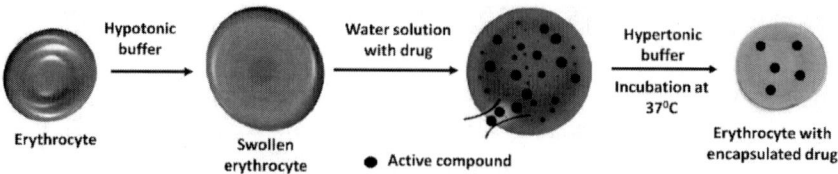

Figure 6. Schematic illustration of hypotonic pre-swelling procedure (adapted according to Kostić 2015).

3.1.4. Hypotonic Dialysis

Method of hypotonic dialysis for encapsulation of enzymes and lipids in erythrocytes was used for the first time in 1977 by Deloach and Ihler (1977). In this procedure, an isotonic buffered suspension of the erythrocytes with hematocrit ranging from 70-80% is placed in a dialysis tube, and then immersed in 10-20 times higher volume of hypotonic buffer with constant stirring for about 2 hours. The tonicity of the cell suspension in the dialysis tube is restored by adding hypertonic buffer to the surrounding medium or by replacing the hypotonic buffer with an isotonic one (Danon 1961). Biologically active compound intended for encapsulation can be dissolved in isotonic buffer inside the dialysis tube at the beginning of the procedure or it can diffuse to dialysis bag from surrounding hypotonic buffer. Cell-encapsulating drug manufactured by this method has life span equal to life span of normal cells in circulation (Magnani et al. 1998). This method has high encapsulation efficiency (30 to 50%), high cell recovery (70 to 80%), and the possibility of automation and on-line monitoring of the process variables (Patel et al. 2008). However, the process is time consuming and demands special equipment. Magnani and co-workers have developed the method for encapsulation of "non-diffusible drugs" (polar substances which do not diffuse through intact membrane) in human erythrocytes (Magnani et al. 1998). This method includes two sequential hypotonic dilutions of erythrocytes, followed by erythrocyte condensation with hemofilter, addition of drug and final erythrocyte resealing step (Figure 7). The described method was used for encapsulation of L- asparaginase (Kravtzoff et al. 1990), recombinant human erythropoietin (Garin, López and Luque 1997), homodinucleotide active against human immunodeficiency virus and herpes simplex virus (Rossi et al. 2001a), antiretroviral drug zidovudine (Briones, Colino and Lanao 2010) and dexamethasone (Rossi et al. 2004; Annese et al. 2005; Castro et al. 2006; 2007; Bossa et al. 2008; 2013). Apparatus developed by EryDel S.p.A (Urbino, Italy) for dexamethasone sodium phosphate encapsulation by hypotonic dialysis was approved in Europe as a medical device (Biagiotti et al. 2011). Its improved version, called EryDex System version 3.2.0, was recently released as a novel CE marked, fully automated and user friendly equipment for dexamethasone sodium phosphate entrapment in autologous erythrocytes (Mambrini et al. 2017). This concept of dexamethasone encapsulation has already been proved as effective treatment for several inflammatory diseases, such as obstructive pulmonary disease (Rossi et al. 2001b), cystic fibrosis (Rossi et al. 2004), various inflammatory bowel diseases (Annese et al. 2005; Bossa et al. 2008; Castro et al. 2006; 2007) and ataxia telangiectasia (Chessa et al. 2014).

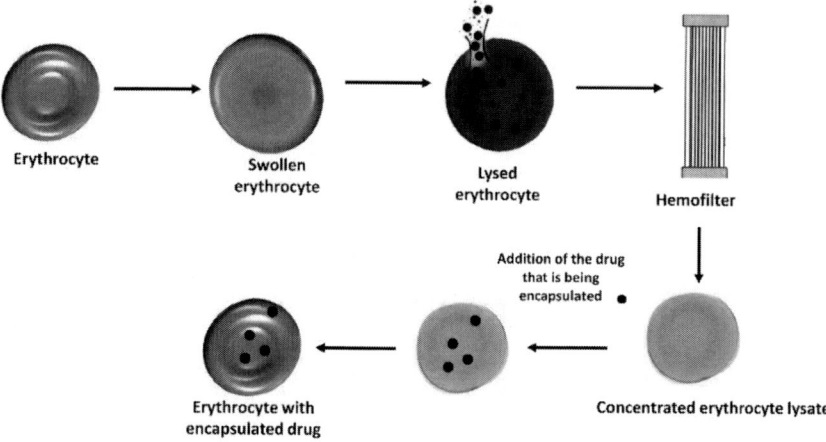

Figure 7. Schematic illustration of hypotonic dialysis procedure (adapted according to Kostić 2015).

4. ERYTHROCYTES UNDER HYPOTONIC CONDITIONS: MODELING CONSIDERATIONS

Currently, osmosis-based drug encapsulation within erythrocyte membranes is studied mainly experimentally, whereas related theoretical models are scarce (Ge et al. 2017). Although based on the same principle, aforementioned encapsulation methods (see section 3) have various operating procedures, causing large differences in the quantity of loaded drugs, often without provision of the most optimal processing parameters (Ge et al. 2017). In this section, we have described a set of equations developed to simulate the erythrocyte behavior under hypotonic conditions and potential drug encapsulation process.

Erythrocyte response under hypotonic conditions includes the following successive sub-bioprocesses: (1) erythrocyte swelling, (2) lifetime of the lipid structural integrity and the rearrangements of trans-membrane protein band 3, (3) the reversible hemolytic pore formation and hemoglobin release to surrounding solution; accumulation of drug inside the cells. Duration of the membrane relaxation per single cell depends on the contributions of three sub-processes: (1) time for cell swelling $t_{sw\,eq} \leq$ ~100 s, (2) membrane lifetime $\tau \in (0, t_H)$ (where t_H is the hemolytic time) and (3) time for hemoglobin (Hb) release and drug loading from already formed hemolytic pore during successive open-closed state changes $t_R = n_j(t_{o\,eq} + t_{c\,eq})$ (where $n_j = 1 - 8$ is the number of repeated open/closed cycles for human erythrocytes, $t_{o\,eq}$~0.27 s is the hole opening time period, $t_{c\,eq}$~0.26 s is the hole closing time period for human erythrocytes, and the Hb released time is $t_{R\,eq} < 5\,s$ (Zade-Oppen 1998; Pribush, Meyerstein and Meyerstein 2002). The time $t_{c\,eq}$ is the time required for the membrane to undergo repeated stretching driven by differential solvent pressure between the intracellular region and external medium. Zade-Oppen (1998) observed repetitive erythrocyte "jumps" during Hb release after erythrocyte swelling. Every jump corresponds to the repeated hemolytic hole opening period. The relaxation time for cell swelling under hypotonic conditions depends on the solution tonicity. Pribush, Meyerstein and Meyerstein (2002) reported that the swelling time for human erythrocytes is equal to 15 s for corresponding external solution made by isotonic solution and water in the ratio 1:5. When the solution tonicity increases up to the ratio 1:1.5 the swelling time increases up to 75 s. The rearrangement time of band 3 molecules for human erythrocytes under hypotonic conditions is: ~500 s under tonicity of 5.2 mM Na_2HPO_4 at 21°C and ~1200 s under tonicity of 5.2 mM Na_2HPO_4 at 21°C (Golan and Veatch 1980).

4.1. Erythrocyte Swelling

Erythrocyte swelling is induced by solvent in-flow driven by the total osmotic pressure difference between the intracellular region and external medium $\Delta P_T(t_{sw}) = P_{in}(t_{sw}) - P_{out}(t_{sw})$ (where $P_{in}(t_{sw})$ is the total pressure within the intracellular region and $P_{out}(t_{sw})$ is the pressure within the external medium. After the in-flow of solvent, the in-flow of Na$^+$ cations and out-flow of K$^+$ cations follow. Delano (1995) proposed van't Hoff's Law for the pressure difference. Interior and exterior pressures for single cells are expressed as:

$$P_{in}(t_{sw}) = RT\phi_{in}C_{in}(t_{sw})$$
$$P_{out}(t_{sw}) = RT\phi_{out}C_{out}(t_{sw}) \tag{1}$$

where R is the universal gas constant, T is temperature, ϕ_{in} and ϕ_{out} are the average intracellular and external osmotic coefficients respectively; $C_{in}(t_{sw})$ and $C_{out}(t_{sw})$ are the intracellular and external solute concentration respectively. If the volume of external solution V_{ext} is different by many orders of magnitude than the volume of single erythrocyte $V_e(t_{sw})$, the external solute concentration is unchanging, $C_{out}(t_{sw}) \sim const$ as well as the external pressure $P_{out}(t_{sw}) \sim const$. The total pressure difference decreases during swelling caused by the intracellular solute concentration decrease. Equilibrium cell swelling state that accomplishes at $t_{sw} = t_{sw\ eq}$ has been described using Young-Laplace equation (Delano 1995):

$$dA_e(t_{sw\ eq})\gamma = dV_e(t_{sw\ eq})\Delta P_T(t_{sw\ eq}) \tag{2}$$

where $A_e(t_{sw\ eq}) = 4R_e(t_{sw\ eq})^2 \pi$ is the surface of swollen erythrocyte, γ is the surface tension of the lipid bilayer, $V_e(t_{sw\ eq}) = \frac{4}{3}R_e(t_{sw\ eq})^3 \pi$ is the volume of swollen erythrocyte.

The rate of cell swelling depends on the external solution tonicity and the viscoelasticity of the membrane. It is expressed by Pajic-Lijakovic (Pajic-Lijakovic 2015a; Pajic-Lijakovic and Milivojevic 2017) as:

$$r_{sw} = \frac{\Delta V_e}{t_{sw}} \tag{3}$$

where r_{sw} is, the erythrocyte swelling rate and ΔV_e is the erythrocyte volume increase. Aging of cells and various diseases influence their rheological behavior. Aged erythrocytes become stiffer and fragile (Nash and Meiselman 1983). The membrane viscoelasticity depends on: (1) the viscoelasticity of the spectrin-actin cortex, (2) the viscoelasticity of the bilayer, (3) the bilayer-cortex coupling and spatial distribution of band 3 molecules (Pajic-Lijakovic 2015b). Pajic-Lijakovic and Milivojevic (2014) proposed constitutive stress-strain model for the viscoelasticity of softer cells such as erythrocytes under thermal fluctuations within two regimes. Short-time regime corresponds to the time scale of milliseconds while the long-time regime corresponds to seconds. The model has been formulated as:

$$\sigma(t) = B\, D_t^{-(\alpha+1)}\varepsilon(t) + \eta_{effC} D_t^\alpha\, \varepsilon(t) + \eta_{effL} D_t^{2\alpha}\, \varepsilon(t)$$
$$\text{for regime 1} \tag{4}$$
$$\sigma(t) = G_{sc}\varepsilon(t) + \eta_{effC} D_t^\alpha\, \varepsilon(t) + \eta_{effL} D_t^{2\alpha}\, \varepsilon(t) \text{ for regime 2}$$

where $\sigma(t)$ is the membrane stress, $\varepsilon(t)$ is the membrane strain, G_{sc} is the cortex shear modulus, η_{effC} is the cortex effective modulus, B is the cortex rearrangement modulus, η_{effL} is the bilayer effective modulus, while operators: $D_t^{-(\alpha+1)}(\cdot)$, $D_t^\alpha(\cdot)$, and $D_t^{2\alpha}(\cdot)$ are fractional derivatives. The fractional derivative of a function $f(t)$ is equal to $D_t^\alpha(f(t)) = \frac{d^\alpha}{dt^\alpha}(f(t))$. We used Caputo's definition of the fractional derivative (Podlubny 1999) as follows: $D_t^\alpha(f(t)) = \frac{1}{\Gamma(1-\alpha)}\frac{d}{dt}\int_0^t \frac{f(t')}{(t-t')^\alpha}dt'$ (where t is independent variable -time and $\Gamma(1-\alpha)$ is the gamma function). The order of fractional derivative α is $0 < \alpha < 1$ represents the damping coefficient of the membrane structural changes. Higher values of the model parameters G_{sc}, η_{effc}, B, and α corresponds to stiffer and the more fragile cortex.

4.2. The Membrane Structural Changes after Erythrocyte Swelling and before Formation of the Hemolytic Hole

After erythrocyte swelling, structural integrity of the lipid bilayer is maintained during the membrane lifetime period. This long-time period corresponds to the band 3 mobile fraction increase. The value of band 3 mobile fraction in the erythrocyte before swelling is small, up to 1%. Change of erythrocyte shape and volume during swelling induces significant dissociation of the low affinity complexes of band 3, and band 3 molecules form clusters. Clusters can perturb their state by thermal fluctuations of the membrane. Excited clusters: (1) can be disintegrated to smaller ones or (2) can change their packing state from closed packing to ring like structure (Pajic-Lijakovic et al. 2010; Pajic-Lijakovic 2015a). Ring like structure of band 3 represents the reversible hemolytic pore (Sato, Yamakose and Suzuki 1993; Pajic-Lijakovic et al. 2010). Helfrich type bending free energy functional has been modified to consider the structural ordering of band 3 molecules (Shlomovitz and Gov 2008; Kabaso et al. 2011; Pajic-Lijakovic 2015b; Pajic-Lijakovic and Milivojevic 2017):

$$E_B(\phi) = \int \frac{1}{2} \kappa_{eff}(\phi)(H - \phi \bar{H}_s)^2 d^2 r \tag{5}$$

where $\phi = \phi(r, \tau)$ is the local volume fraction of inclusions such as band 3 molecules in the erythrocyte membrane, $\kappa_{eff}(\phi)$ is the effective bending modulus of the lipid bilayer, H is the local mean curvature, $\bar{H}_s$ is the curvature induced by conformations of the surrounding spectrin filaments. The effective bending modulus of the lipid bilayer could be correlated with the bilayer effective modulus η_{effL} (eq. 4). It is expressed by Shlomovitz and Gov (2008) as:

$$\kappa_{eff}(\phi) = \kappa(1-\phi) + \kappa'\phi \tag{6}$$

where κ is the bending modulus of the lipid bilayer without inclusions, κ' is the contribution of inclusions to the bending modulus. Shlomovitz and Gov (2008) described the lateral diffusion of band 3 molecules as:

$$\frac{\partial \phi(\tau)}{\partial \tau} = D_B \nabla^2 \phi(\tau) + \lambda \nabla \left(\phi(\tau) \nabla \left(\frac{\delta E_B(\phi(\tau))}{\delta \phi(\tau)} \right) \right) \tag{7}$$

where ∇ is the derivative along the space, λ is the band 3 mobility and D_B is the band 3 diffusion coefficient equal to $D_B = \frac{k_B T}{\lambda}$.

4.3. Hemoglobin Release and Drug Loading under Hypotonic Conditions

Hemoglobin (Hb) release and drug loading are accomplished simultaneously through hemolytic hole. The loading/release time period consist of simultaneous opening and closing time periods of the hole. A single opening time period is $t_o \in [0, t_{o\ eq}]$ while the single closing time period is $t_c \in [0, t_{c\ eq}]$. The number of repeated open-closed periods of the reversible hemolytic hole depends on external solution tonicity and cell morphology.

The driving force for Hb release is the Hb pressure difference equal to (Delano 1995; Pajic-Lijakovic 2015a):

$$\Delta P_{Hb}(t_o, t_R) = P_{in\ Hb}(t_o, t_R) - P_{out\ Hb}(t_o, t_R) \tag{8}$$

where t_R is the Hb release time, $P_{in\ Hb}(t_o, t_R)$ is the Hb pressure within the intracellular region, $P_{out\ Hb}(t_o, t_R)$ is the Hb pressure within the external medium. Interior and exterior pressures of Hb for single cells are expressed as:

$$P_{in\ Hb}(t_o, t_R) = RT\phi_{in\ Hb}C_{in\ Hb}(t_o, t_R)$$
$$P_{out\ Hb}(t_o, t_R) = RT\phi_{out\ Hb}C_{out\ Hb}(t_o, t_R) \qquad (9)$$

where $\phi_{in\ Hb}$ and $\phi_{out\ Hb}$ are the average Hb intracellular and external osmotic coefficients respectively; $C_{in\ Hb}(t_o, t_R)$ and $C_{out\ Hb}(t_o, t_R)$ are the intracellular and external Hb concentration respectively.

The Hb mass flow through the hemolytic holes during single opening cycle is (Pajic-Lijakovic et al. 2010; Pajic-Lijakovic 2015a):

$$Q_{Hb}(t_o, t_R) = k_{Hb}\Delta C_{Hb}(t_o, t_R)A_H(t_o, t_R) \qquad (10)$$

where k_{Hb} is the coefficient of mass transfer through the hemolytic hole, $A_H(t_o, t_R)$ is the surface of the reversible hemolytic hole. When $t_o \to t_{o\ eq}$, the released amount of Hb $m_{Hb}(t_R) = \int_0^{t_{oeq}} Q_{Hb}(t_o, t_R)dt_o$ causes the cell volume decrease and consequently decrease of the membrane stretching state which leads to the hemolytic hole closing, i.e $A_H \to 0$. Human erythrocyte loses 6% of its swollen volume during single opening time period of the hemolytic hole (Zade-Oppen 1998).

The driving force for drug loading is the drug pressure difference equal to:

$$\Delta P_D(t_o, t_R) = P_{out\ D}(t_o, t_R) - P_{in\ D}(t_o, t_R) \qquad (11)$$

where $P_{in\ D}(t_o, t_R)$ is the drug pressure within the intracellular region, $P_{out\ D}(t_o, t_R)$ is the drug pressure within the external medium. Interior and exterior pressures of drug for single cells are expressed as:

$$P_{in\ D}(t_o, t_R) = RT\phi_{in\ D}C_{in\ D}(t_o, t_R)$$
$$P_{out\ D}(t_o, t_R) = RT\phi_{out\ D}C_{out\ D}(t_o, t_R) \qquad (12)$$

where $\phi_{in\,D}$ and $\phi_{out\,D}$ are the average drug intracellular and external osmotic coefficients respectively; $C_{in\,D}(t_o, t_R)$ and $C_{out\,D}(t_o, t_R)$ are the intracellular and external drug concentration respectively.

The drug mass flow through the hemolytic pores during single opening cycle is:

$$Q_D(t_o, t_R) = k_D \Delta C_D(t_o, t_R) A_H(t_o, t_R) \tag{13}$$

where k_D is the coefficient of drug mass transfer through the hemolytic hole. When $t_o \to t_{o\,eq}$, the loaded amount of drug is equal to $m_D(t_R) = \int_0^{t_{oeq}} Q_D(t_o, t_R) dt_o$.

Described modelling consideration provides better understanding and quantification of the mechanisms of pore formation on erythrocyte membrane with an aim of drug entrapment and optimization of the processing parameters for osmosis-based drug encapsulation (Ge et al. 2017).

5. ERYTHROCYTE MEMBRANE BASED AND ERYTHROCYTE MEMBRANE IMPROVED DDS: PHYSICO-CHEMICAL CHARACTERIZATION AND BIOLOGICAL ACTIVITY

Although the term erythrocyte carrier stands for both intact erythrocyte and erythrocyte membrane, from a historical point of view, firstly it was related to the erythrocyte membrane, so called ghost, as a delivery system for enzymes (Ihler, Glew, and Schnure 1973). At first, the studies revealed that resulting erythrocyte ghosts (resultant envelopes or cell-like structures) prepared by fast hemolysis process from erythrocytes are osmotically competent too, it was suggested that substances like soluble enzymes might be loaded within them (Ihler, Glew, and Schnure 1973). Due to inevitable hemoglobin loss during erythrocyte ghosts preparation procedures based on pronounced hemolysis (which led to their reduced survival in circulation), as well as membrane alteration (which led to their recognition by macrophages), erythrocyte ghosts were first investigated as possible carriers for targeted drug delivery in diseases associated with the mononuclear phagocyte system (Dale et al. 1979; Eichler et al. 1986). A few studies on targeting erythrocyte ghosts to other cells, such as T cells and peritoneal macrophages have been reported (Chiarantini et al. 1995; DeLoach and Droleskey 1986). Even though the first membrane derivatives were short-circulating compared to intact erythrocytes, in theory, they were regarded as the systems that could reach target sites otherwise inaccessible to erythrocytes. These investigations led to the development of new derivatives of erythrocyte membranes (ghosts), exosome-like fragments of erythrocytes, i.e., vesicles called "nanoerythrosomes" (Moorjani et al. 1996, Lejeune et al. 1994, Désilets et al. 2001). As the blood cell based biomimetic carriers, nanoerythrosomes exhibit many favorable properties such as very high surface area-to-volume ratio (~ 80 times higher than parent erythrocyte), and could be as small as 100 nm (Gupta, Patel and Ahsan 2014). Production of vesicles from erythrocyte ghosts with a diameter of few hundred nanometers is based on colloid chemistry principles and physics: filtration, extrusion, sonication or electric pulses (Pouliot et al. 2002; Gupta, Patel and Ahsan 2014; Deák et al. 2015). Depending on the percentage of cells recovered after the removal of intracellular components, in general one erythrocyte can be fragmented into 4000–5000 nanoerythrosomes (Gupta, Patel and Ahsan 2014). Drug can be loaded by one of the described osmosis based procedures (see section 3), (Gupta, Patel and Ahsan 2014, Mishra and Jain 2003) or conjugated onto nanoerythrosomal surfaces, as shown in the case of conjugated daunorubicin and pyrimethamine (Agnihotri and Jain 2013, Lejeune et al. 1994). Regarding the route of administration, nanoerythrosomes have been investigated as intravenous, intra-peritoneal, subcutaneous and inhalational drug carriers (Zhang 2016; Gupta, Patel and Ahsan 2014, Dong et al. 2017).

The composition and properties of the resulting nanoerythrosomes are comparable to the original cell membrane (Pouliot et al. 2002; Banerjee and Singh 2013), if the process used for their preparation is controlled;

thus, an optimal combination of lysis media, processing temperature and sizing technique is required to develop a stable nanoerythrosomes formulation (Schwoch and Passow 1973; Lieber and Steck 1989; Gupta, Patel and Ahsan 2014). Deák et al. (2015) demonstrated preparation of very stable vesicles derived from erythrocyte membranes (with mean diameter of 200 nm and zeta potential of -42 mV), due to preserved intrinsically present membrane protein and carbohydrate components. More specifically, although steps during ghost preparation (such as centrifugation and washing out with lysis buffers) remove most of the peripheral proteins, optimized pH and temperature can help in preserving the amount and quality of integral proteins, as confirmed by TEM images of the ghosts (Deák et al. 2015). The large number of homogeneously distributed integral proteins on the membrane surface of nanoerythrosomes revealed by TEM analysis, can serves as a quality control of the nanoerythrosomes stock dispersion before further processing (Deák et al. 2015). Freshly prepared ghost membranes are large sheets, their lateral size is about 2-4µm, while fracture surfaces are randomly speckled with intramembrane protein particles (typical size less than 10 nm) (Deák et al. 2015). Similarly, Gupta, Patel and Ahsan (2014) produced nanoerythrosomes formulation spherical in shape, with an average size of 154.1 ± 1.31 nm, stable for 3 weeks when stored at 4°C, and drug loading efficiency of 48.76 ± 2.18%. Kuo et al. (2016) assessed colloidal properties of nanoerythrosomes prepared from bovine erythrocytes and compared them with the liposomes as conventional DDS. It was shown that nanoerythrosomes prepared by erythrocyte ghosts sonication for 15 min, gave stable dispersion of nanoerythrosomes with an average size of 110 nm having unilamellar membrane of thickness ~4.5 nm (Kuo et al. 2016). Remarkably, the biconcave disc-like shape of erythrocytes was also exhibited when nanoerythrosomes were placed in hypertonic buffers and unlike typical liposomes, nanoerythrosomes had excellent colloidal stability in both buffer as well as in serum at room temperature; moreover, these erythrocyte membrane based-nanostructures can be decorated with fluorescent or other markers, solutes can be encapsulated in their cores, and they can be targeted to specifically bind to mammalian cells (Kuo et al. 2016).

Although promising results were obtained after initial *in vitro* studies of anti-tumor effects of prototype derivatives of erythrocyte membranes loaded with cytotoxic agents (Lejeune et al. 1994; Moorjani et 1996; Villa et al. 2016), expected long life span of these DDS *in vivo* was not demonstrated. However, various glycans and proteins on the erythrocyte membrane surface make encapsulated cargos more stable under physiological conditions in comparison to the free form of cargo (Huang et al. 2016). For instance, in one recent study, nanoerythrosomes loaded with anti-malarial agent were cleared in rats within a few hours, but slightly slower than free drug (Agnihotri et al. 2015). Furthermore, nano-sized erythrocyte ghosts prepared from Sprague dawley rats demonstrated successful encapsulation of sodium tanshinone IIA sulfonate (STS), widely used agent in treatment of cardiovascular diseases for arteries expansion and blood flow speed up; compared with STS injection, these STS-nano-ghosts (average size 156 nm with polydispersity index of 0.045) prolonged the drug release both *in vitro* and *in vivo* and revealed superior repairing outcome on oxidative stress-impaired endothelial cells (Dong et al. 2017).

Recently, alternative strategies regarding the use of erythrocyte membrane nano-derivatives have emerged (Villa et al. 2016). In one of them, erythrocyte membranes cover the synthetic nanoparticles to hinder them from the immune system of the host, so-called "RBC-cloaked" nanoparticles (Hu et al. 2011). In this study, erythrocyte ghosts were isolated after hypotonic lysis and further extruded together with carboxylated PLGA nanoparticles (~70 nm) to obtain the RBC-cloaked particles (Hu et al. 2011). These hybrid biomimetic particles demonstrated longer circulation in comparison to PLGA-based one, and even PEG covered particles (Hu et al. 2011). Erythrocyte membrane-nanoparticles were also able to efficiently deliver a doxorubicin to solid tumor sites for significantly improved tumor growth inhibition compared with conventional free drug treatment (Aryal et al. 2013). The main advantage of these hybrid drug formulations is association of the immunomodulatory properties of natural erythrocyte membrane components with the drug carrying capacity of polymeric nanoparticles (Luk 2016). Luk and co-authors (2015) have thoroughly examined the interfacial features of such hybrid systems: they showed successful right-side-out membrane cloaking approach applied to negatively charged nanoparticles between 65 and 340 nm (Luk et al. 2015). Furthermore, they revealed that these hybrid DDS are completely shielded by lipid membranes, and are stabilized by surface glycans and negatively charged sialic acid residues; this structural reorganization of nano-sized erythrocyte membrane prevents positively charged nanoparticles coverage (Luk et al. 2015). In addition to targeted drug delivery, erythrocyte membrane-cloaked carriers can be also used as a platform for vaccination (Hu et al. 2013) and toxin absorption (Fang et al. 2015). Other studies demonstrated that such erythrocyte membrane hybrid formulations can be also produced using inorganic core (Fang et al. 2013) or gold nanocages (Piao et al. 2014). Red blood cell membrane-cloaked gold nanocages were presented to provide enhanced photothermal tumor ablation versus non-cloaked counterparts (Piao et al. 2014).

Autologous rat red blood cell ghosts prepared by hypotonic pre-swelling method without reducing their size down to the nano-scale, demonstrated successfully targeted delivery of cytokines IL-1ß to the sites of inflammation, i.e., wound infections; this ghost based DDS improved the pharmacokinetic profiles of IL-1 β by increasing its half-life, reducing its clearance, and increasing the deposition of the drug in the liver, spleen and lungs (Berikkhanova et al. 2016). Microbiological and cytological analysis of wound exudates in this study showed a significant speeding up of healing processes in a group of animals treated with a local injection of IL-1 β and ceftriaxone encapsulated into erythrocyte ghosts in comparison with the animals treated either with a local or intramuscular injection of free drugs (Berikkhanova et al. 2016). Erythrocyte membranes with preserved structure prepared by complete hemoglobin removal from human erythrocytes appeared as an excellent gene delivery system as well (Huang et al. 2016). In comparison to the commercial Roche gene transfection reagent and the polyethylenimine derivative, this erythrocyte membrane based system displayed much higher transfection efficiency and minimal cytotoxicity, not only in the highly transfectable cell line (i.e., human embryonic kidney cells), but also in many hard-transfect cell lines, such as human umbilical cord mesenchymal stem cells (Huang et al. 2016).

One more interesting approach related to the erythrocyte membrane based systems development is small modification in the membranes that allow them to be controlled by external stimuli, as demonstrated by Hsiesh et al. (2015). Namely, Hsiesh et al. (2015) produced carriers (average size 1-2 μm) consisting of a camptothecin-loaded mouse erythrocyte membrane shell with a liquid core of perfluoride-n-pentane (C5F12), through a process based on hypotonic treatment and sonication. Short (3 min) high intensity focused ultrasound insonation induced violent vaporization of C5F12 in these erythrocyte ghosts based derivatives, consequently impairing the integrity of the membrane and release of the drug; generated physical explosion of droplets in these DDS further promoted drug distribution into the interstitial region of a tumor and tumor cells death, by disrupting local vascular endothelial junctions. These generated microbubbles could serve as an imaging contrast agent because of their high acoustic impedance too (Hsiesh et al. 2015).

Furthermore, isolated erythrocyte membranes without reducing the size down to the nano-scale also successfully served as a template for fabrication of layer-by-layer (LbL) microcapsules, drug delivery systems which can finely tune the release profile of encapsulated substance (Shaillender et al. 2011). In comparison to conventionally prepared LbL microcapsules, ghosts based LbL microcapsules provided simpler mean for the preparation of loaded LbL microcapsules, eliminating the core dissolution and post-loading of bioactive agents; furthermore, through this approach, the shell made of polyelectrolyte layers regulates the release profiles of the encapsulated molecules by the number of added layers, concomitantly protecting the erythrocyte ghosts from decomposition as well as the bioactivity of encapsulated drugs or proteins (Shaillender et al. 2011). Further, layer-by-layer assembly of polyelectrolytes, which are non-immunogenic, can cover antigenic determinants expressed on erythrocyte membranes (Mansouri et al. 2011); thus, the abovementioned strategy of erythrocyte membrane templated microcapsules encourages the use of even xenogeneic, i.e., animal erythrocytes as constitutes of DDS. Next section will provide in detail an overview of complexity of research and prerequisite investigational steps toward the potential use of animal erythrocytes as drug delivery vehicles, conducted by our research group.

6. CASE STUDY: DEVELOPMENT OF ANIMAL ERYTHROCYTE GHOSTS BASED DRUG CARRIERS

Autologous erythrocytes seem to be very effective systems for targeted delivery and prolonged release of various drugs (Villa et al. 2016; Pierigè et al. 2017; Millán, Bravo and Lanao 2017; Han, Wang and Liu 2018). The fact that several protocols for the infusion of active substances encapsulated into erythrocytes are currently in the clinical trial stage illustrates the colossal biomedical importance of this field of research (Pierigè et al. 2017). Since biotechnological methods provide immunogenicity attenuation through modification of the cell membrane (Mansouri et al. 2011; Cerda-Cristerna et al. 2012), the possibility of heterologous erythrocytes use as universal carriers of drugs exists. This includes even xenogeneic (animal) erythrocytes, which are already of great importance as delivery vehicle of therapeutic and/or diagnostic compounds in preclinical studies (Pierigè et al. 2017).

However, suitable technology permitting the use of animal erythrocytes as universal DDS has not been developed so far. Such technology would be of great importance, especially considering the facts that the use of autologous blood erythrocytes for personalized treatment is expensive and that other available sources of human erythrocytes, from voluntary blood donors, are scarce. Due to exceptional biological properties and to a great extent universal structure of erythrocyte membranes regardless of the type of origin (see section 2), in this section, we emphasize the feasibility of preparation of erythrocyte membranes from bovine and porcine slaughterhouse blood as potential carriers for prolonged delivery of anti-inflammatory drug, dexamethasone-sodium phosphate. Erythrocytes from slaughterhouse waste blood are available in enormous quantities; this way the application of slaughterhouse blood erythrocytes prepared as DDS is economically justified and harmonized with the recommendations for implementing more sustainable and higher value practices in recovery of slaughterhouse blood as industry by- product (Lynch et al. 2017). All necessary research steps in engineering and characterization of erythrocyte membranes isolated from bovine and porcine erythrocytes, to act as potential drug delivery systems *in vitro*, are described in this section.

In our studies (Kostić et al. 2014; Bukara et al. 2016; Drvenica et al. 2016) slaughterhouse blood was taken from jugular vein of Swedish Landrace swine and Holstein-Friesian cattle. Blood was collected in a sterile glass bottles with 3.8% sodium-citrate as an anticoagulant, and transported at ambient temperature. Porcine and bovine erythrocytes were precipitated by blood centrifugation at 2450×g for 20 min at 4°C. Plasma and leucocytes were carefully discarded by vacuum aspiration. The precipitated erythrocytes were resuspended in an isotonic phosphate buffered saline, pH 7.2-7.4 (PBS, 0.8% saline buffered with 10 mM sodium phosphate) and washed twice by centrifugation. As described above, the establishment of optimal osmolarity (hypotonic) conditions in line with the specific osmotic properties of erythrocytes allows optimized isolation of red blood cell membranes and consequent encapsulation of active substances within the membranes. Thus, the initial step in our research was to examine the osmotic properties of erythrocytes acquired from bovine and porcine slaughterhouse blood in term of their osmotic resistance and swelling degree.

Prior to the examination of osmotic properties, the analysis of basic hematological characteristics of bovine and porcine erythrocytes isolated from slaughterhouse blood showed that the mean values of erythrocyte and hemoglobin concentration, hematocrit, as well as the values of MCV (mean corpuscular volume), MCH (mean corpuscular hemoglobin) and MCHC (mean corpuscular hemoglobin concentration) did not differ significantly from the reference values in healthy animals (Kostić et al. 2014). This finding suggests that basic parameters of erythrocyte quality are not altered by sodium citrate that has been used as an anticoagulant and during the plasma protein removal and the preparation of packed erythrocytes for erythrocyte ghosts manufacturing. Additionally, it was confirmed by mechanical fragility test, that bovine and porcine red blood cells isolated from slaughterhouse blood did not exhibit a significant degree of mechanically induced hemolysis; in other words, these erythrocytes when handled properly, as described above, may be used as an initial biomaterial to produce erythrocyte ghosts (Kostić et al. 2015).

It is well known that mammalian erythrocytes differ in many properties: size, volume and shape, lipid membrane composition, composition and structural organization of transmembrane and cytoskeletal proteins, enzymatic activity, ionic composition, ATP and other metabolites (Jain 1993; Harvey 2008). Each of these features affects the osmotic properties of erythrocytes to a greater or lesser extent. Nevertheless, data on the osmotic properties of animal erythrocytes are very limited and inconsistent. Thus, Jain (1993) claims that there is a linear relationship between the size of the erythrocytes and their osmotic resistance. According to this claim, bovine erythrocytes, which are smaller in size than porcine erythrocytes, are expected to be less osmotically resistant compared to porcine erythrocytes. On the other hand, our results are comparable with the results obtained by Matsuzawa and Ikarashi (1979), as well as Brzezińska-Slebodzińska (2003) and Johnstone and colleagues (2004) (Kostić et al. 2014; Kostić et al. 2015), indicating that bovine erythrocytes (although cells smaller in size) are more osmotically resistant than porcine erythrocytes. Our results showed that 50% of hemolysis of porcine erythrocytes is caused by 118 mM sodium chloride solution (0.69% NaCl solution), while in bovine erythrocyte samples 50% hemolysis was achieved in 108 mM solution of sodium chloride (0.60% NaCl solution) (Kostić et al. 2014). For the sake of comparison, according to the data published by Matsuzawa and Ikarashi (1979), 50% of hemolysis (H_{50}) was determined in 0.51% and 0.47% NaCl solution for porcine and bovine erythrocytes, respectively. In the study of Johnstone and colleagues (2004), the H_{50} value was determined in 0.56% NaCl solution for porcine and 0.48% NaCl for bovine erythrocytes. Increased osmotic fragility of porcine erythrocytes may be a consequence of oxidative damage induced by the transportation of animals from farm to slaughterhouse and/or the treatment of animals in slaughterhouse, as suggested by other authors (Adenkola et al. 2010; Mota-Rojas et al. 2012). It is known that among investigated mammalian erythrocytes so far, porcine erythrocytes are the most sensitive to oxidative stress induced by free radicals (Brzezińska-Slebodzińska 2003). In addition to the study by Jain (1993), to the best authors' knowledge there are no other literature data on the degree of swelling of bovine and porcine erythrocytes. In order to define an optimal buffer system (hypoosmotic) to induce controlled hemolysis of erythrocytes, while preserving the structure of their membrane, the degree of hemolysis and swelling of bovine and porcine erythrocytes in Na-phosphate/NaCl buffers of different concentrations (pH 7.2-7.4) were measured using two methods: microhematocrit method (according to Vitvitsky et al. (2000) and flow cytometry (according to the modified method of Piagnerelli et al. (2007)). The two methods employed in our studies yielded consistent results regarding the osmotic fragility of the investigated erythrocytes (Kostić et al. 2014; Kostić et al. 2015), confirming that porcine erythrocytes are osmotically more fragile than bovine erythrocytes. Furthermore, the flow cytometry method, through the osmotic swelling test, confirmed the existence of osmotically different erythrocyte fractions in samples isolated from bovine and porcine slaughterhouse blood (Kostić et al. 2015). This was preliminary indicated by derivation analysis of the data obtained by conventional osmotic fragility test (Kostić et al. 2014). As already known, bimodal cell-size distribution detected by flow cytometry is typical for biconcave cells, such as erythrocytes when the cells are placed in isotonic medium (van den Bos et al. 1992). Since the erythrocytes placed in hypotonic environment acquire spherical shape, the obtained erythrocyte size distribution by flow cytometry (conducted under hypotonic conditions) reveal the existence of osmotically different erythrocyte fractions in samples isolated from bovine and porcine slaughterhouse blood. Based on this result and the data in the literature reporting on human erythrocytes (Sternberg et al. 2011), a different amount of encapsulated drug per individual erythrocyte ghosts is to be expected if the hypotonic hemolysis based method is used for drug encapsulation (Kostić et al. 2014; Kostić et al. 2015).

In our studies (Kostić et al. 2014; Drvenica et al. 2016; Bukara et al. 2016) the isolation of erythrocyte ghosts, that would contain the amount of hemoglobin as low as possible, was performed by hemolysis process in which the selected hypotonic buffers (chosen according to the osmotic fragility analysis) were introduced gradually. This process of gradual hypotonic hemolysis can be carried out under sterile conditions, it is simple and cost-effective, because it only requires a reactor vessel in which the hemolysis takes place, a mixing system and a peristaltic pump. Due to the possibility of scaling up the process, it is designed in such a way that only low-priced buffer systems (Na-phosphate / NaCl buffers) are used, without nutrient addition (Kostić 2015). Additives could increase the quality of the obtained erythrocyte ghosts (Millán et al. 2004a), but also increase the overall cost of the process. Based on the results of a detailed examination of the osmotic properties of bovine and porcine erythrocytes from slaughterhouse blood, in our laboratory, hemolysis of the high volume of erythrocytes (100 ml, hematocrit (Hct) 60%, continuously mixed on the orbital shaker at 320 rpm) was performed using 35 mM Na-phosphate/NaCl buffer gradually introduced by flow rate of 300 ml/h for 30 min. These process parameters enabled more than 90% of hemolysis for both types of erythrocytes (Kostić et al. 2014). Plotting the extent of hemolysis versus time resulted in sigmoidal curves (Figure 8A), demonstrating that hemolysis, i.e., the extracellular hemoglobin, was first detected after 3 min for both erythrocyte samples tested. However, 50% of hemolysis was reached at the 14th min for bovine and 10th min in the case of porcine erythrocytes. Bovine erythrocytes were completely hemolysed after 27 min, which corresponded to buffer concentration of 74 mM. The gradual hemolysis for porcine erythrocytes was ended at the 21st min, which corresponded to buffer concentration of 80 mM. These results confirmed the previously presented findings that bovine erythrocytes are more osmotically resistant than porcine ones, regardless of whether the erythrocytes are suddenly or gradually exposed to hypotonic solution. The process progression was also monitored by timeline reduction in the number of erythrocytes, as depicted in Figure 8B. The number of cells undergoing hemolysis decreased in a cascade manner, which was more pronounced in the case of bovine erythrocytes, confirming the existing difference in susceptibility to osmotic lysis between the bovine and porcine red blood cells. The sequence of the appearance of erythrocyte ghosts was verified by phase contrast microscopy (Figure 8C and D). It was observed that most of the erythrocytes were converted to ghosts, i.e., intact membranes without hemoglobin at the end of the process. The resulting ghosts were washed four times with PBS and separated by centrifugation at 3220 × g and 4°C during 40 min.

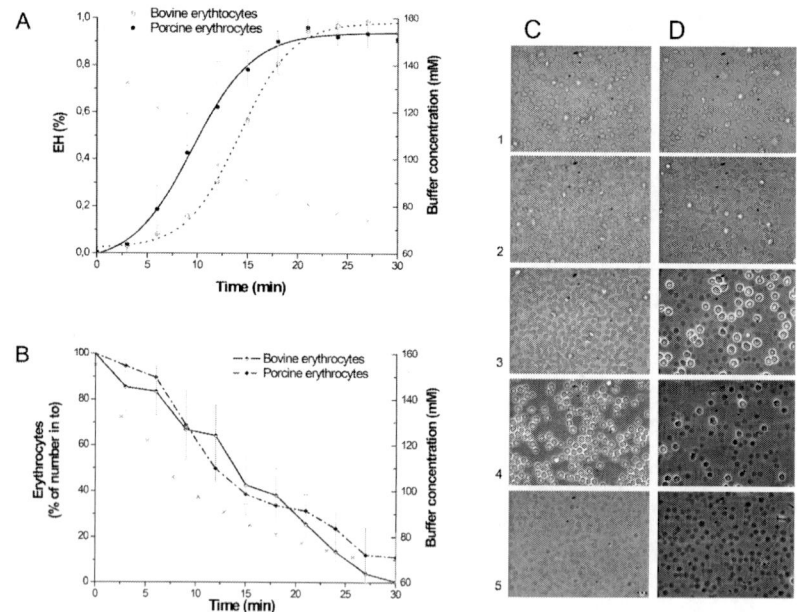

Figure 8. Gradual hypotonic hemolysis of bovine and porcine erythrocytes. The time course of hemoglobin release (A); points – mean ± SD of three samples; lines – fitting curves. The time dependent changes in erythrocyte number (B); points – mean ± SD of three samples; (x) – calculated values of gradual tonicity decrease. Phase contrast microscopy analysis of morphological changes of erythrocytes from bovine (C) and porcine (D) slaughterhouse blood and appearance of erythrocyte ghosts during gradual hypotonic hemolysis; micrographs are obtained in the following time points/corresponding sodium-phosphate/NaCl buffer concentrations: (1) 4 min/130 mM, (2) 6 min/120 mM, (3) 9 min/105 mM, (4) 18 min/84 mM and (5) 26 min/75 mM; magnification 400×. (Reprinted from Colloid Surf B., 122, Kostić et al. 2014, *Erythrocyte membranes from slaughterhouse blood as potential drug vehicles: Isolation by gradual hypotonic hemolysis and biochemical and morphological characterization*, 250–259. Copyright ©2014, with permission from Elsevier.)

It is important to characterize the isolated erythrocyte membranes of bovine and porcine erythrocytes in terms of morphological and biochemical properties which could have an impact on the diffusion and partition coefficient of the potentially encapsulated active substance (Kostić et al. 2014). Based on a review of literature, it is known that in the case of some polymeric drug delivery systems, the encapsulated drug is released by desorption from the surface and diffusion from the inner volume; in general, the manner of the drug release depends a lot on size, roughness and the specific surface of the material used for encapsulation (Biondi et al. 2008). Thus, in terms of morphology, the topographic characteristics are important to be analyzed - shape, size, and roughness of the isolated empty bovine and porcine erythrocyte ghosts. The morphological analysis of the erythrocyte ghosts of both animal species by field emission scanning electron microscopy (FE-SEM) revealed a significant distortion from the erythrocyte shape, and change in the texture of a surface with pronounced invaginations (Kostić et al. 2014). Echinocyte like morphology that was noted in both porcine and bovine erythrocyte ghosts had already been demonstrated in human ATP-depleted erythrocytes, and in human erythrocyte ghosts obtained by lysis in a hypotonic PBS solution (Harris, Smith and Bell 2001). Results of the size and size distribution measurement by laser diffraction method, in line with obtained data by FE-SEM analysis, indicated that the process of gradual hemolysis led to decrease in size only for 10% in average of the resulting ghosts compared to the initial erythrocytes (Kostić et al. 2014; Bukara et al. 2016). For the sake of comparison, Montes et al. (2008) claimed that the classical hemolysis, so-called "osmotic shock" produce human erythrocyte ghosts with an average diameter three times smaller than the size of the starting erythrocytes.

Although sodium dodecyl sulfate polyacrylamide gel electrophoresis (SDS-PAGE) is considered as "rough" method for determining protein content, it can be extremely useful in assessing the impact of various chemical and physical agents on the overall protein composition of the erythrocyte membrane (Grebowski, Krokosz and Puchala 2013). SDS-PAGE analysis revealed that all the major protein fractions generally found in intact erythrocyte membranes are present in bovine and porcine erythrocyte membranes obtained in our lab by gradual hypotonic hemolysis (Kostić et al. 2014). However, annexin V binding test showed that the erythrocyte membranes of both species exhibit phosphatidylserine in the outer layer of the membrane, indicating that gradual hemolysis induces reorganization in the phospholipid bilayer (Kostić et al. 2014). It has been already shown that the exposure of bovine erythrocytes to oxidative stress causes the partial expression of phosphatidylethanolamine (40%) and phosphatidylserine (30-33%) in the outer layer of the membrane phospholipid double layer (Wali et al. 1987). The presence of phosphatidylserine in the outer layer occurs when erythrocytes are exposed to hypotonic environment (Muzykantov 2010). In addition, osmotic stress caused by the exposure of erythrocytes to hypotonic solutions can cause the formation of "the inside-out" ghosts (Andrade et al. 2004); all the mentioned could be the reasons for the exhibition of phosphatidylserine on the surface of red blood cell membranes in our study. Low level of changes in the distribution of phospholipids and the average size of bovine and porcine erythrocyte membranes isolated by gradual hypotonic hemolysis (Kostić et al. 2014), implies the overall relatively conserved lipid composition of both types of erythrocyte ghosts according to the report by DeLoach and Spates (1988). If isolated erythrocyte ghosts would serve as active substance carriers, the demonstrated structural alteration in the membrane would probably lead to their recognition and takeover by macrophages (Fan et al. 2012). In such a way prepared erythrocyte ghosts offer a greater application potential for targeted delivery of active substances to macrophages and dendritic cells (Kostić et al. 2014).

Cholesterol, which is the key regulator of cell membrane fluidity (through the effect on the "packing" of the lipids in the cell membrane) and the deformability of the membrane (via modulation of the interaction of membrane proteins in the outer part of the cytoskeleton (Sun et al. 2007)), can significantly affect the passage of the active substance and its retention in the erythrocyte membrane. Our results have shown that more than 90% of cholesterol present in the intact bovine and porcine erythrocytes is retained in erythrocyte ghosts resulted from gradual hypotonic hemolysis

(Kostić et al. 2014). Given the preserved size of erythrocyte ghosts, cholesterol and protein content, one can assume that erythrocyte ghosts from slaughterhouse blood could mimic the chemical and structural anisotropic cell membrane environment *in vivo*. Such characteristics are of great importance for the consequent diffusion and partition coefficient of encapsulated drugs within erythrocyte ghosts (Kostić et al. 2014).

In order to demonstrate the application of the process of gradual hypotonic hemolysis, we have used two drugs for encapsulation into the erythrocyte ghosts: dexamethasone sodium phosphate and diclofenac sodium phosphate, as models of steroid and non-steroid anti-inflammatory drugs, respectively (Drvenica et al. 2016; Bukara et al. 2016). For this purpose, 50 mL of washed packed erythrocytes were resuspended in isotonic PBS to a hematocrit of 60%, and poured in a 2 L glass beaker. Afterwards, the hypotonic PBS of 70 mOsm/kg containing specified concentration of drug (Drvenica et al. 2016; Bukara et al. 2016) was introduced gradually by infusion pump with a flow rate of 150 mL/h during 27 min. The ghosts were separated by centrifugation and washed with a hypotonic PBS four times. The remaining relative quantity of hemoglobin, within the erythrocyte membranes, is calculated as described in Kostić et al. (2014). Afterwards, 1 mL of ghosts was annealed in 8 mL of isotonic PBS (30 min, at room temperature (25°C) or 37°C), containing drug at specified concentration (Drvenica et al. 2016; Bukara et al. 2016). Then, the same volume of ghosts was transferred to 8 mL of hypertonic buffer containing the same drug concentration and incubated for 90 min at 25 and 37°C. Finally, the ghost carriers were washed three times using PBS by centrifugation, to wash out the un-entrapped drug. In some experiments sham-encapsulated ghosts (i.e., the erythrocyte membranes under complete loading procedure with no added drug) were needed. These were prepared as described except that the drug aqueous solution was replaced by drug-free buffer solution (Drvenica et al. 2016; Bukara et al. 2016). Compared to the other methods for encapsulation of active substances into erythrocyte membranes described in section 3, one can conclude that the gradual hypotonic hemolysis is based on the principles of several methods. Namely, the process is designed to remove hemoglobin from erythrocytes as much as possible, since this protein can be further used as a source of valuable heme-iron for treatment of iron deficiency (Stojanović et al. 2012; Pravilović et al. 2012). This step of hemoglobin removal is the main feature of the hypotonic hemolysis method in general (see section 3.1.1). The content of hemoglobin in the final dispersion of erythrocyte ghosts largely depends on age and inter-individual variations in the starting erythrocytes (Kostić et al. 2014). To a lesser degree, the content of hemoglobin depends on the number of PBS washing cycles after performed hemolysis. Furthermore, the drug itself, during encapsulation process, can influence the hemoglobin content in the final ghosts: Bukara et al. (2016) demonstrated that through applied encapsulation process by gradual hypotonic hemolysis, diclofenac loaded porcine erythrocyte ghosts retained 3-4 folds more hemoglobin in comparison with the empty erythrocyte ghosts.

Described process of gradual hypotonic hemolysis has the characteristics of a hypotonic dilution by means of a drug added at the beginning of the process with hypotonic saline solutions. However, it is comparable with hypotonic dialysis, since the drug is added in the second phase with hypertonic buffer (see section 3). In addition, gradual hypotonic hemolysis also controls the erythrocyte swelling, which is the main characteristic of the hypotonic pre-swelling method (see section 3.1.3). Thus, the main advantage of the applied gradual hypotonic hemolysis is the precise control of erythrocyte swelling, preventing their burst in the hypotonic environment. This would allow the reversible opening of the hemolytic holes and consequent encapsulation of active substances, followed by incubation in the hypertonic solution (Kostić 2015; Drvenica et al. 2016; Bukara et al. 2016). Also, gradual hypotonic hemolysis does not require expensive specially designed equipment, as it is the case with hypotonic dialysis method (see section 3.1.4).

There are two main analytical aspects to be considered within research and development of new drug delivery systems: the quantification of drug content in the carrier and the quantification of drug that has been released from the carrier (Martín-Sabroso et al. 2013). This means that the procedure for carrier degradation must be established in such a way to provide recovery of the total amount of encapsulated drug. Further, the extracted drug must be quantified in a specific, accurate and reproducible manner (Rivas, Gil-Alegre and Torres-Suárez 2006). Regarding the quantification of a drug that has been liberated from the carrier, the developed analytical procedure must detect very low drug concentrations in the release medium and selectively quantify it in the presence of other components of DDS, which can also be released into the medium (Martín-Sabroso et al. 2013). Due to the complex chemical structure of the investigated erythrocyte ghosts (consisting of lipids, proteins and carbohydrates) as the drug carriers, the prerequisite for our studies was the development of an analytical procedure for the absolute identification and quantification of the encapsulated drug(s). Encapsulated dexamethasone sodium phosphate and diclofenac sodium phosphate were identified in samples based on their mass spectrometry (MS) and MS/MS spectra, compared to the drug standards (Drvenica et al. 2016; Bukara et al. 2016). This analytical method enabled us to differentiate the dephosphorylated form - dexamethasone from dexamethasone sodium phosphate. Dephosphorylated dexamethasone occurs due to the conversion of dexamethasone sodium phosphate encapsulated in erythrocyte carriers (Rossi et al. 2001b; Rossi et al. 2004; Biagiotti et al. 2011). The presence of dephosphorylated drug form, dexamethasone, was not detected in either porcine or bovine erythrocyte ghosts, indicating the complete recovery of the initial drug encapsulated into the erythrocyte ghosts (Drvenica et al. 2016). Apart from unambiguous identification and quantification of the drug encapsulation process, the analytical methods developed in our studies allowed us to optimize the process parameters for encapsulation (initial concentration of the drug, incubation temperature, glutaraldehyde addition), and to monitor the drug release kinetics from the ghost based systems (Kostić 2015). By examining the influence of process parameters on the efficiency of dexamethasone sodium phosphate encapsulation in bovine and porcine erythrocytes membranes, it has been shown that incubation at 37°C has a significant effect on the amount of encapsulated drug in erythrocyte ghosts (Drvenica et al. 2016). Under the same experimental conditions, a much higher amount of encapsulated dexamethasone sodium phosphate was obtained in porcine than in bovine erythrocyte ghosts. This can be explained by the specific composition of phospholipids in bovine erythrocyte membrane along with the influence of liposomal lipid composition (as artificial membrane analogues) on encapsulation and release control of encapsulated drug (Kostić 2015). Namely, in mammals, phosphatidylcholine is generally the most abundant phospholipid in the composition of erythrocyte membranes; however, a deviation from this "rule" is seen in bovine erythrocyte membranes, which are particularly deficient in phosphatidylcholine, but contain higher level of sphingomyelin (Florin-Christensen et al. 2001). Slower release of encapsulated drug from liposomes containing sphingomyelin compared to the liposomes without sphingomyelin has been already shown (Webb et al. 1995). Thus, by establishing an analogy between erythrocyte membranes and liposomes, it is possible to explain the reduced permeability of bovine erythrocyte membranes for dexamethasone sodium phosphate encapsulation compared to porcine erythrocyte membranes. In addition, dexamethasone sodium phosphate encapsulation in both types of erythrocyte ghosts was directly proportional to the increase in drug concentration in the incubation buffer within the concentration range of 0.04-0.12 mg/ml (Drvenica et al. 2016). Obtained data are consistent with the results published by Millán et al. (2008), Hamidi et al. (2007b, 2007c), and Foroozesh et al. (2011), related to the encapsulation of various drugs in human erythrocyte ghosts using hypoosmotic methods. Achieved dexamethasone sodium phosphate encapsulation efficiency in porcine erythrocyte ghosts (13-14%) in our study (Drvenica et al. 2016) is similar to those obtained by encapsulating various active compounds (drugs, enzymes, proteins, polysaccharides, DNA) into the human erythrocyte ghosts by hypoosmotic procedures (Millán et al. 2008; Staedtke et al. 2010; Shaillender et al. 2011). In our other study–sodium diclofenac revealed encapsulation efficiency of 37% in porcine erythrocyte ghosts (Bukara et al. 2016). Low encapsulation efficiency that has been shown in the case of bovine erythrocyte ghosts (2-3%) in our study (Drvenica et al. 2016) was not considered as a negative result. Dexamethasone sodium phosphate is hydrophilic drug and during the encapsulation procedure, it tends to diffuse from the external environment (buffer with the dissolved drug) into the inner "aqueous" medium of erythrocyte ghosts.

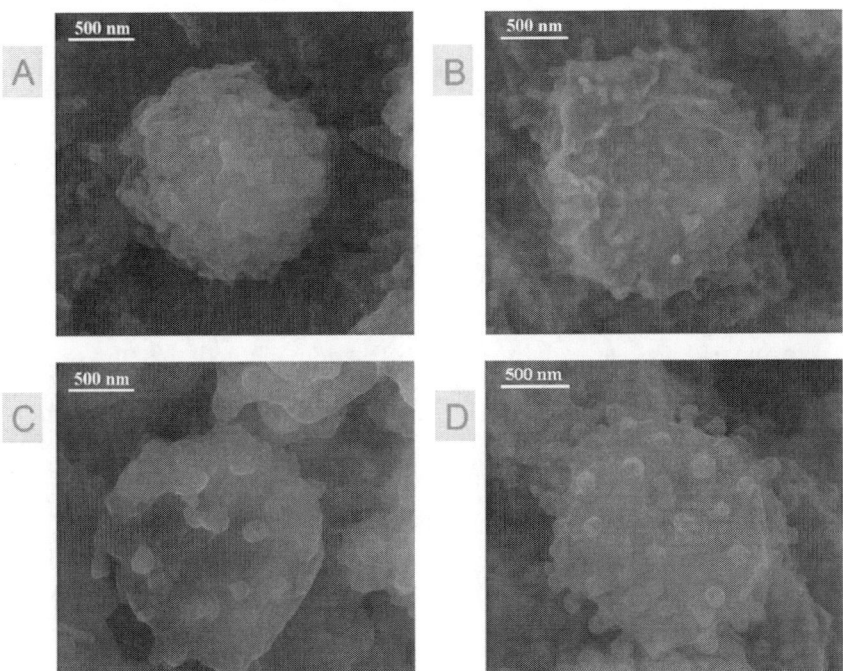

Figure 9. Scanning electron micrographs of (A) sham encapsulated bovine erythrocyte ghosts, (B) dexamethasone sodium phosphate encapsulated bovine erythrocyte ghosts, (C) sham encapsulated porcine erythrocyte ghosts, and (D) dexamethasone sodium phosphate encapsulated porcine erythrocyte ghosts. (This material is reproduced with permission of John Wiley & Sons, Inc. from Drvenica et al. 2016, *Biotechnology Progress*, Copyright ©2016 American Institute of Chemical Engineers.)

Including the lower encapsulation efficiency obtained in the case of bovine erythrocyte ghosts, it can be assumed that the diffusion resistance of bovine erythrocyte membrane to dexamethasone sodium phosphate is higher in comparison to the diffusion resistance of porcine erythrocyte membrane (Drvenica et al. 2016). In addition, the results of low encapsulation efficiency of dexamethasone sodium phosphate in bovine ghosts were comparable with the data published by Kim et al. (2009) on the entrapment of antisense oligonucleotide in human erythrocyte ghosts by procedure involving hypotonic and isotonic phosphate buffers.

Conversely, Sternberg et al. (2011) have shown that the efficacy of encapsulation of FITC-labeled bovine serum albumin into the human erythrocyte ghosts (without hemoglobin) is almost 97%. In this study, phosphate buffers have also been used in the procedure for encapsulation of FITC-labeled bovine serum albumin. Given that Kim and co-workers (2009) showed that the use of other buffers in encapsulation procedure could improve the efficiency of encapsulation, a possible explanation for the results obtained in our study, could be that the use of phosphate buffer is not suitable for bovine erythrocyte ghosts resealing; nevertheless, these speculations merit further investigations. As previously stated, phosphate buffers are cost-effective, non-toxic and safe.

We have demonstrated by laser diffraction method that the size of erythrocyte ghosts with and without dexamethasone sodium phosphate is approximately the same for both types of animal erythrocyte ghosts (Kostić et al. 2015b). This result was confirmed by FE-SEM and atomic force microscopy (AFM) (Drvenica et al. 2016). FE-SEM micrographs showed the minimal differences in shape, size, and topology of sham encapsulated erythrocyte ghosts vs. dexamethasone sodium phosphate encapsulated into erythrocyte ghosts; however, these alterations were more pronounced in the case of porcine erythrocyte ghosts than in bovine ones (Figure 9). Additionally, FE-SEM and AFM gave consistent results on the surface roughness of bovine and porcine erythrocyte ghosts with encapsulated dexamethasone sodium phosphate (Figure 10). The drug encapsulation in bovine ghosts led only to a small decrease of root mean square (RMS) of surface roughness in comparison to the control bovine erythrocyte ghosts, from 17.2 ± 1.5 nm to 15.9 ± 2.8 nm ($p > 0.05$). In the case of porcine erythrocyte ghosts, RMS values for surface roughness were 30.0 ± 5.4 nm and 34.2 ± 7.5 nm for control and dexamethasone sodium phosphate encapsulated porcine erythrocyte ghosts, respectively ($p > 0.05$) (Drvenica et al. 2016). The AFM analysis showed that addition of drug in the gradual hypotonic hemolysis procedure has no evident effect on the morphology of produced erythrocyte carriers. However, the AFM analysis confirmed the existence of a significant difference in morphology between the bovine and porcine erythrocyte ghosts (for both controls and with encapsulated drug, p

<0.05), which can greatly affect the characteristics i.e., behavior of these two investigated types of erythrocyte ghosts as dexamethasone sodium phosphate carriers (Drvenica et al. 2016).

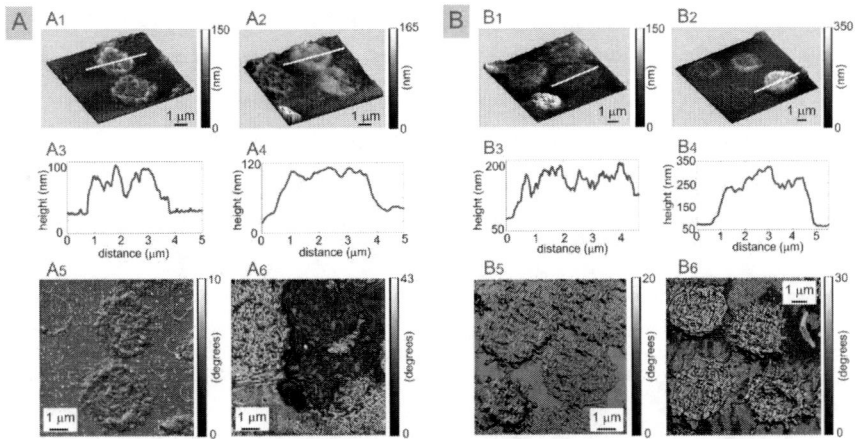

Figure 10. (A) AFM analysis of dexamethasone sodium phosphate encapsulation procedure impact on morphology of bovine (A1) Sham encapsulated erythrocyte ghosts, (A2) dexamethasone sodium phosphate encapsulated erythrocyte ghosts. (B) AFM analysis of dexamethasone sodium phosphate encapsulation procedure impact on morphology of porcine (B1) Sham encapsulated erythrocyte ghosts; (B2) dexamethasone sodium phosphate DexP encapsulated erythrocyte ghosts. Parts A1, A2, B1, and B2 show three-dimensional topographies. Parts A3, A4, B3, and B4 depict the height profile along the lines denoted in parts A1, A2, and B1, B2, respectively. Parts A5, A6, B5, and B6 represent AFM phase images obtained simultaneously with the topographic images. (This material is reproduced with permission of John Wiley & Sons, Inc. from Drvenica et al. 2016, *Biotechnology Progress*, Copyright ©2016 American Institute of Chemical Engineers.)

Encapsulation of dexamethasone sodium phosphate and its release kinetics significantly differed between the types of erythrocyte ghost samples and between the samples of the same species, depending on the residual hemoglobin content (Drvenica et al. 2016). In contrast to porcine cell membrane carriers, bovine carriers have shown multiphase release kinetics of encapsulated dexamethasone sodium phosphate. For both types of erythrocyte ghost carriers, the existence of a *lag* phase shows that the process of the drug release from the ghosts involves, apart from simple diffusion, some structural entities from the cell membrane (Kostić 2015). It is well known that drug release kinetics from erythrocyte carriers depends on the size and polarity of the encapsulated substances (Shaillender et al. 2011). In general, three different manners of drug release are considered: 1) drug release is performed by rapid diffusion through the membrane, as shown in the case of lipophilic drug primakine (Talwar and Jaind 1992), 2) drug release is accomplished by cell membrane lysis, as shown in the case of enalaprilat (Hamidi et al. 2001), and tramadol (Foroozesh et al. 2011), 3) drug release profile is a combination of the first two ways, as shown for isoniazid (Jain, Jain and Dixit 1995) and erythropoietin (Garin et al. 1997).

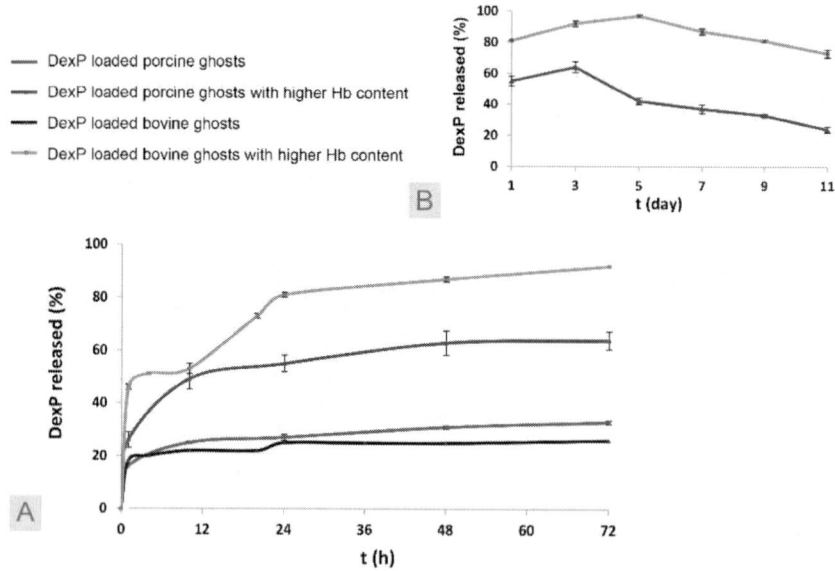

Figure 11. The release profiles of dexamethasone sodium phosphate (DexP) from bovine and porcine erythrocyte ghost carriers. The release profiles in first 72 h (A) and from Day 1 up to Day 11 (B). Values are mean ±SD (n = 3). (This material is reproduced with permission of John Wiley & Sons, Inc. from Drvenica et al. 2016, *Biotechnology Progress*, Copyright ©2016 American Institute of Chemical Engineers.)

As presented in Figure 11A, dexamethasone sodium phosphate release profile from red blood cell membrane carriers had greater drug efflux in the case of both types of ghosts (bovine and porcine) with a higher hemoglobin content (during the same experimental time) compared with the ghosts with a lower residual hemoglobin content (Drvenica et al. 2016).

Furthermore, the effect of residual hemoglobin was more pronounced in the case of bovine erythrocyte ghosts in comparison to the porcine ones. This fact supports the theory that the release of drug is accelerated by the release of hemoglobin from erythrocyte carriers (Hamidi et al. 2001; Foroozesh et al. 2011). The residual hemoglobin in the ghosts appeared as a new quality parameter necessary to be controlled in order to standardize the production of bovine and porcine erythrocyte ghosts based DDS (Drvenica et al. 2016). Since biochemical analysis in our studies showed very similar structure of bovine and porcine erythrocyte ghosts to the initial erythrocytes, comparable transport characteristics through isolated membranes as in intact erythrocyte membranes can be expected (Kostić 2015). Besides, demonstrated differences in the release profiles of dexamethasone sodium phosphate from bovine and porcine carriers indicate the existence of various efflux transporters, which mediate the active efflux of the drug encapsulated within the erythrocyte membranes, as some authors have already suggested (Hamidi et al. 2007c; Harisa, Ibrahim and Alnazi 2011). In our study, prolonged release of dexamethasone sodium phosphate from bovine (during 5 days) and porcine erythrocyte ghosts (during 3 days) was achieved (Drvenica et al. 2016). In the case of diclofenac sodium encapsulated within porcine ghosts, similar release profile during four days was obtained (Bukara et al. 2016). An observed phenomenon of the declining trend of dexamethasone sodium phosphate release after 3 days in the case of porcine and 5 days in the case of bovine erythrocyte ghosts (Figure 11B) is most likely the result of drug instability. This is caused by interaction of some of the structural components of the complex assembly of erythrocyte membranes with the drug under the experimental conditions used in the drug release test (e.g., solubilization of the drug by membrane present fatty acids, etc.). The assumption that the amount of drug released in the medium is reduced due to its dephosphorylation and conversion into dexamethasone was rejected after UHPLC/-HESI-MS / MS analysis (Drvenica et al. 2016). The decline in the amount of drug released in the medium has already been described in the case of tramadol encapsulated in human erythrocytes, where the decreasing trend in drug release was observed after 5 days (Foroozesh et al. 2011).

Bearing in mind the demonstrated features of drug encapsulated bovine and porcine erythrocyte ghosts, it seems that they could have a future in drug delivery, including the field of nanomedicines, as starting material in the production of nanoerythrosomes (Drvenica et al. 2016, Bukara et al. 2016). In other words, our data on these animal drug loaded erythrocyte ghosts have been encouraging enough to merit further *in vitro* and *in vivo* investigation.

CONCLUSION

Only 20 years ago, the erythrocyte membranes were merely used as a model system for studying various cell membrane-related phenomena, such membrane composition and organization or membrane transport properties, as well as for the comparative proteomic and lipidomic analyses in health and disease, leading to improved understanding of disease mechanisms and/or identification of new diagnostic and therapeutic methodologies. The possibility of engineering erythrocyte membranes by encapsulation of drugs, and their capacity to act as a cellular bio-derived drug delivery system (DDS) *per se* or part of hybrid DDS (in conjunction with synthetic nanoparticles), represents a fundamental advancement in the way erythrocytes are currently used. This chapter addresses the main features of such erythrocyte membrane based DDS, their advantages and drawbacks, which principally arises from their intrinsic biological/ physiological species related properties. Intriguing application of erythrocyte membranes as DDS is grounded on the methods of transient opening of pores across them. The pores are large enough to be traversed by externally added molecules of drug, while retaining the possibility to mimic the chemical and structural anisotropic environment of *in vivo* cell membranes. In this chapter, four such osmosis based procedures have been described, placing emphasis on their feasibility, complexity, possibility to scale-up and convenience for research/clinical use. Although there are some general recommendations regarding operating parameters for drug encapsulation, experimental procedures given in literature differ from one another, causing large differences in the quality of final ghost drug carriers, e.g., final amount of drug loaded. Because of the discrepancies, in this chapter we provided a set of equations as a potential tool to better understand and quantify the mechanisms of pore formation on erythrocyte membrane under hypo-osmotic conditions, and consequent optimization of drug loading. We have given an overview of the most recent achievements in production and application of erythrocyte membrane based DDS, offering many benefits compared to free-form drug: prolonged release and consequent reduction of dosage frequency, targeted delivery to specific body districts, encapsulated substance toxicity reduction, and if autologous erythrocytes membranes are used for nanoparticles covering, avoidance of detection of synthetic nanoparticles by immune system. Since animal erythrocyte membranes are already used in preclinical investigations, with tendency for more extensive application as universal drug carriers owing to the emerging bioengineering approaches. In this chapter we have presented our results on complex development and characterization of prolonged drug delivery system based on bovine and porcine erythrocyte ghosts, considering the differences between erythrocytes derived from these two readily available animal blood samples.

ACKNOWLEDGMENT

This work was supported by Ministry of Education, Science and Technological Development, Republic of Serbia (Project No. III46010).

REFERENCES

Adenkola, Adeshina Yahaya, Joseph O. Ayo, Anthony K.B. Sackey, Alexander B. Adelaiye. 2010. "Erythrocyte osmotic fragility of pigs administered ascorbic acid and transported by road for short-term duration during the harmattan season". *African Journal of Biotechnology* 9:226-233.

Agnihotri, Jaya, and Narendra Kumar Jain. 2013. "Biodegradable Long Circulating Cellular Carrier for Antimalarial Drug Pyrimethamine". *Artificial Cells, Nanomedicine, and Biotechnology* 41 (5): 309-314. doi:10.3109/21691401.2012.743901.

Agnihotri, Jaya, Shubhini Saraf, Sobhna Singh, and Papiya Bigoniya. 2015. "Development and Evaluation of Anti-Malarial Bio-Conjugates: Artesunate-Loaded Nanoerythrosomes". *Drug Delivery and Translational Research* 5 (5): 489-497. doi:10.1007/s13346-015-0246-y.

Andolfo, Immacolata, Roberta Russo, Antonella Gambale, and Achille Iolascon. 2016. "New Insights on Hereditary Erythrocyte Membrane Defects". *Haematologica* 101 (11): 1284-1294. doi:10.3324/haematol.2016.142463.

Andrade, Cristina, Lígia A.M Barros, Maria Celiana Pinheiro Lima, and Edwin G. Azero. 2004. "Purification and Characterization of Human Hemoglobin: Effect of the Hemolysis Conditions". *International Journal of Biological Macromolecules* 34 (4): 233-240. doi:10.1016/j.ijbiomac.2004.05.003.

Annese, Vito, Anna Latiano, Luigina Rossi, Giovanni Lombardi, Bruno Dallapiccola, Sonia Serafini, Giancarlo Damonte, Angelo Andriulli, and Mauro Magnani. 2005. "Erythrocytes-Mediated Delivery of Dexamethasone in Steroid-Dependent IBD Patients-A Pilot Uncontrolled Study". *The American Journal of Gastroenterology* 100 (6): 1370-1375. doi:10.1111/j.1572-0241.2005.41412.x.

Aoki, Takahiko. 2017. "A Comprehensive Review of Our Current Understanding of Red Blood Cell (RBC) Glycoproteins". *Membranes* 7 (4): 56. doi:10.3390/membranes7040056.

Arese, Paolo, Franco Turrini, and Evelin Schwarzer. 2005. "Band 3/Complement-Mediated Recognition and Removal of Normally Senescent and Pathological Human Erythrocytes". *Cellular Physiology and Biochemistry* 16 (4-6): 133-146. doi:10.1159/000089839.

Aryal, Santosh, Che-Ming J. Hu, Ronnie H. Fang, Diana Dehaini, Cody Carpenter, Dong-Er Zhang, and Liangfang Zhang. 2013. "Erythrocyte Membrane-Cloaked Polymeric Nanoparticles for Controlled Drug Loading and Release". *Nanomedicine* 8 (8): 1271-1280. doi:10.2217/nnm.12.153.

Berikkhanova, Kulzhan, Rustam Omarbaev, Alexandr Gulyayev, Zarina Shulgau, Dilbar Ibrasheva, Gulsim Adilgozhina, Shynggys Sergazy, Zhaxybay Zhumadilov, and Sholpan Askarova. 2016. "Red Blood Cell Ghosts as Promising Drug Carriers to Target Wound Infections". *Medical Engineering & Physics* 38 (9): 877-884. doi:10.1016/j.medengphy.2016.02.014.

Bhaskaran, Shyamala and S.S. Dhir. 1995. Resealed erythrocytes as carriers of salbutamol sulphate. *Indian Journal of Pharmaceutical Sciences.* 57(6): 240-242

Biagiotti, Sara, Maria Filomena Paoletti, Alessandra Fraternale, Luigia Rossi, and Mauro Magnani. 2011. "Drug Delivery by Red Blood Cells". *IUBMB Life* 63 (8): 621-631. doi:10.1002/iub.478.

Biondi, Marco, Francesca Ungaro, Fabiana Quaglia, and Paolo Antonio Netti. 2008. "Controlled Drug Delivery in Tissue Engineering". *Advanced Drug Delivery Reviews* 60 (2): 229-242. doi:10.1016/j.addr.2007.08.038.

Bird, J., R. Best, and D.A. Lewis. 1983. "The Encapsulation of Insulin in Erythrocytes". *Journal of Pharmacy and Pharmacology* 35 (4): 246-247. doi:10.1111/j.2042-7158.1983.tb02921.x.

Bossa, Fabrizio, Anna Latiano, Luigia Rossi, Mauro Magnani, Orazio Palmieri, Bruno Dallapiccola, and Sonja Serafini et al. 2008. "Erythrocyte-Mediated Delivery Of Dexamethasone In Patients With Mild-To-Moderate Ulcerative Colitis, Refractory To Mesalamine: A Randomized, Controlled Study". *The American Journal of Gastroenterology* 103 (10): 2509-2516. doi:10.1111/j.1572-0241.2008.02103.x.

Bossa, Fabrizio, Vito Annese, Maria Rosa Valvano, Anna Latiano, Giuseppina Martino, Luigia Rossi, and Mauro Magnani et al. 2013. "Erythrocytes-Mediated Delivery of Dexamethasone 21-Phosphate in

Steroid-Dependent Ulcerative Colitis". *Inflammatory Bowel Diseases*, 1 doi:10.1097/mib.0b013e3182874065.

Brenner, Jacob S., Daniel C. Pan, Jacob W. Myerson, Oscar A. Marcos-Contreras, Carlos H. Villa, Priyal Patel, and Hugh Hekierski et al. 2018. "Red Blood Cell-Hitchhiking Boosts Delivery of Nanocarriers to Chosen Organs by Orders of Magnitude". *Nature Communications* 9 (1). doi:10.1038/s41467-018-05079-7.

Briones, Elsa, Clara I. Colino, and José M. Lanao. 2010. "Study of the Factors Influencing the Encapsulation of Zidovudine in Rat Erythrocytes". *International Journal of Pharmaceutics* 401 (1-2): 41-46. doi:10.1016/j.ijpharm.2010.09.006.

Brunori, Maurizio, Saverio G. Condo, Andrea Bellelli, and Bruno Giardina. 1982. "Hemoglobins from Wistar Rat: Crystallization of Components and Intraerythrocytic Crystals". *European Journal of Biochemistry* 129 (2): 459-463. doi:10.1111/j.1432-1033.1982.tb07071.x.

Brzezińska-Slebodzińska, Ewa. 2003. "Species differences in the susceptibility of erythrocytes exposed to free radicals in vitro". *Veterinary Research Communication* 27:211-217.

Bugarski, Branko and Nebojsa Dovezenski and Hemofarm Koncern. 2000. *Verfahren zur Herstellung von Hemoglobin [Process for the preparation of hemoglobin]*, Deutsches Patentamt DE 19707508.

Bukara, Katarina, Ivana Drvenica, Vesna Ilić, Ana Stančić, Danijela Mišić, Borislav Vasić, Radoš Gajić, Dušan Vučetić, Filip Kiekens, and Branko Bugarski. 2016. "Comparative Studies on Osmosis Based Encapsulation of Sodium Diclofenac in Porcine and Outdated Human Erythrocyte Ghosts". *Journal of Biotechnology* 240: 14-22. doi:10.1016/j.jbiotec.2016.10.017.

Castro, M., L. Rossi, B. Papadatou, F. Bracci, D. Knafelz, M.I. Ambrosini, and A. Calce et al. 2007. "Long-Term Treatment with Autologous Red Blood Cells Loaded With Dexamethasone 21–Phosphate in Pediatric Patients Affected By Steroid-Dependent Crohn Disease". *Journal of Pediatric Gastroenterology and Nutrition* 44 (4): 423-426. doi:10.1097/mpg.0b013e3180320667.

Castro, Massimo, Daniela Knafelz, Luigia Rossi, Maria Irene Ambrosini, Bronislava Papadatou, Giovanni Mambrini, and Mauro Magnani. 2006. "Periodic Treatment with Autologous Erythrocytes Loaded With Dexamethasone 21-Phosphate for Fistulizing Pediatric Crohn's Disease". *Journal of Pediatric Gastroenterology and Nutrition* 42 (3): 313-315. doi:10.1097/01.mpg.0000188006.59128.47.

Cerda-Cristerna, Bernardino Isaac, Sophie Cottin, Luca Flebus, Amaury Pozos-Guillén, Héctor Flores, Ernst Heinen, and Olivier Jolois et al. 2012. "Poly (2-Dimethylamino Ethylmethacrylate)-Based Polymers to Camouflage Red Blood Cell Antigens". *Biomacromolecules* 13 (4): 1172-1180. doi:10.1021/bm300127f.

Chambers, Elizabeth, and Samir Mitragotri. 2004. "Prolonged Circulation of Large Polymeric Nanoparticles by Non-Covalent Adsorption on Erythrocytes". *Journal of Controlled Release* 100 (1): 111-119. doi:10.1016/j.jconrel.2004.08.005.

Chessa, Luciana, Vincenzo Leuzzi, Alessandro Plebani, Annarosa Soresina, Roberto Micheli, Daniela D'Agnano, and Tullia Venturi et al. 2014. "Intra-Erythrocyte Infusion Of Dexamethasone Reduces Neurological Symptoms In Ataxia Teleangiectasia Patients: Results Of A Phase 2 Trial". *Orphanet Journal of Rare Diseases* 9 (1): 5. doi:10.1186/1750-1172-9-5.

Chiarantini, Laura, Luigia Rossi, Alessandra Fraternale, and Mauro Magnani. 1995. "Modulated Red Blood Cell Survival By Membrane Protein Clustering". *Molecular and Cellular Biochemistry* 144 (1): 53-59. doi:10.1007/bf00926740.

Dale, G.L., W. Kuhl, and E. Beutler. 1979. "Incorporation of Glucocerebrosidase into Gaucher's Disease Monocytes in Vitro." *Proceedings of the National Academy of Sciences* 76 (1): 473-475. doi:10.1073/pnas.76.1.473.

Danielyan, Kristina, Kumkum Ganguly, Bi-Sen Ding, Dmitriy Atochin, Sergei Zaitsev, Juan-Carlos Murciano, Paul L. Huang, Scott E. Kasner, Douglas B. Cines, and Vladimir R. Muzykantov. 2008. "Cerebrovascular Thromboprophylaxis in Mice by Erythrocyte-Coupled Tissue-

Type Plasminogen Activator". *Circulation* 118 (14):1442-1449. doi:10.1161/circulationaha.107.750257.

Danon, David. 1961. "Osmotic Hemolysis by a Gradual Decrease in The Ionic Strength Of The Surrounding Medium". *Journal of Cellular and Comparative Physiology* 57 (2): 111-117. doi:10.1002/jcp.1030570208.

Deák, Róbert, Judith Mihály, Imola Cs. Szigyártó, András Wacha, Gábor Lelkes, and Attila Bóta. 2015. "Physicochemical Characterization Of Artificial Nanoerythrosomes Derived From Erythrocyte Ghost Membranes". *Colloids and Surfaces B: Biointerfaces* 135: 225-234. doi:10.1016/j.colsurfb.2015.07.066.

Delano, Michael D. 1995. "Simple Physical Constraints in Hemolysis. *Journal of Theoretical Biology* 175 (4): 517-524. doi:10.1006/jtbi.1995.0159.

DeLoach, J.R., and R. Droleskey. 1986. "Preparation of Ovine Carrier Erythrocytes: Their Action and Survival". *Comparative Biochemistry and Physiology Part A: Physiology* 84 (3): 441-445. doi:10.1016/0300-9629(86)90344-0.

DeLoach, John R. 1985. "Hypotonic dialysis encapsulation in erythrocytes of mammalian species" *Biblioteca Haematologica* 51:1–6.

DeLoach, John R., and George Spates E. 1988. "A comparison of membrane lipid content of normal and carrier-erythrocytes from cattle". *Italian Journal of Biochemistry* 37:386-391.

Deloach, John, and Garret Ihler. 1977. "A Dialysis Procedure for Loading Erythrocytes with Enzymes and Lipids". *Biochimica Et Biophysica Acta (BBA) - General Subjects* 496 (1): 136-145. doi:10.1016/0304-4165(77)90121-0.

DeLoach, J.R., R.L. Harris, and G.M. Ihler. 1980. "An Erythrocyte Encapsulator Dialyzer Used In Preparing Large Quantities of Erythrocyte Ghosts and Encapsulation of a Pesticide in Erythrocyte Ghosts". *Analytical Biochemistry* 102 (1): 220-227. doi:10.1016/0003-2697(80)90342-5.

Désilets, J., A. Lejeune, J. Mercer, C. Gicquaud. 2001. "Nanoerythrosomes, a new derivative of erythrocyte ghost: IV. Fate of reinjected nanoerythrosomes." *Anticancer Research* 21(3B):1741-1747.

Dong, Xiaoting, Yawei Niu, Yi Ding, Yuemin Wang, Jialan Zhao, Wei Leng, and Linghao Qin. 2017. "Formulation and Drug Loading Features of Nano-Erythrocytes". *Nanoscale Research Letters* 12 (1). doi:10.1186/s11671-017-1980-5.

Drvenica, Ivana T., Katarina M. Bukara, Vesna Lj. Ilić, Danijela M. Mišić, Borislav Z. Vasić, Radoš B. Gajić, Verica B. Đorđević, Đorđe N. Veljović, Aleksandar Belić, and Branko M. Bugarski. 2016. "Biomembranes from Slaughterhouse Blood Erythrocytes as Prolonged Release Systems for Dexamethasone Sodium Phosphate". *Biotechnology Progress* 32 (4): 1046-1055. doi:10.1002/btpr.2304.

Eichler, H.G., W. Schneider, G. Raberger, S. Bacher, and I. Pabinger. 1986. "Erythrocytes as Carriers for Heparin". *Research in Experimental Medicine* 186 (6): 407-412. doi:10.1007/bf01852193.

"EP0929317A2 - *Polyethyleneglycol Conjugated Nanoerythrosomes, Method Of Making Same and Use Thereof* - Google Patents". 2019. Patents.Google.Com. https://patents.google.com/patent/EP0929317A2/en.

Fan, Wen, Wei Yan, Zushun Xu, and Hong Ni. 2012. "Erythrocytes Load Of Low Molecular Weight Chitosan Nanoparticles As A Potential Vascular Drug Delivery System". *Colloids and Surfaces B: Biointerfaces* 95: 258-265. doi:10.1016/j.colsurfb.2012.03.006.

Fang, Ronnie H., Brian T. Luk, Che-Ming J. Hu, and Liangfang Zhang. 2015. "Engineered Nanoparticles Mimicking Cell Membranes for Toxin Neutralization". *Advanced Drug Delivery Reviews* 90: 69-80. doi:10.1016/j.addr.2015.04.001.

Fang, Ronnie H., Che-Ming J. Hu, Kevin N.H. Chen, Brian T. Luk, Cody W. Carpenter, Weiwei Gao, Shulin Li, Dong-Er Zhang, Weiyue Lu, and Liangfang Zhang. 2013. "Lipid-Insertion Enables Targeting Functionalization of Erythrocyte Membrane-Cloaked Nanoparticles". *Nanoscale* 5 (19): 8884. doi:10.1039/c3nr03064d.

Favretto, M.E., J.C.A. Cluitmans, G.J.C.G.M. Bosman, and R. Brock. 2013. "Human Erythrocytes as Drug Carriers: Loading Efficiency and

Side Effects of Hypotonic Dialysis, Chlorpromazine Treatment and Fusion With Liposomes". *Journal of Controlled Release* 170 (3): 343-351. doi:10.1016/j.jconrel.2013.05.032.

Florin-Christensen, J., C.E. Suarez, M. Florin-Christensen, M. Wainszelbaum, W.C. Brown, T.F. McElwain, and G.H. Palmer. 2001. "A Unique Phospholipid Organization in Bovine Erythrocyte Membranes". *Proceedings of the National Academy of Sciences* 98 (14): 7736-7741. doi:10.1073/pnas.131580998.

Foroozesh, Mahshid, Mehrdad Hamidi, Adbolhossein Zarrin, Soliman Mohammadi-Samani, and Hashem Montaseri. 2011. "Preparation and In-Vitro Characterization of Tramadol-Loaded Carrier Erythrocytes for Long-Term Intravenous Delivery". *Journal of Pharmacy and Pharmacology* 63 (3): 322-332. doi:10.1111/j.2042-7158.2010. 01207.x.

Gardos, G. 1953. "Akkumulation de Kalium Onen Durch Menschiche Blutkorperchen," *Acta Physiologica Hungarica* 6(2):191-199.

Garin, Marina Inmaculada, Rosa María López, and José Luque. 1997. "Pharmacokinetic properties and in-vivo biological activity of recombinant human erythropoietin encapsulated in red blood cells". *Cytokine* 9 (1): 66-71. doi:10.1006/cyto.1996.0137.

Ge, Duobiao, Lili Zou, Chengpan Li, Sen Liu, Shibo Li, Sijie Sun, and Weiping Ding. 2017. "Simulation of the Osmosis-Based Drug Encapsulation in Erythrocytes". *European Biophysics Journal* 47 (3): 261-270. doi:10.1007/s00249-017-1255-1.

Georgieva, Radostina, Sergio Moya, Edwin Donath, and Hans Bäumler. 2004. "Permeability And Conductivity of Red Blood Cell Templated Polyelectrolyte Capsules Coated with Supplementary Layers". *Langmuir* 20 (5): 1895-1900. doi:10.1021/la035779f.

Golan, D.E., and W. Veatch. 1980. "Lateral Mobility of Band 3 in the Human Erythrocyte Membrane Studied By Fluorescence Photobleaching Recovery: Evidence for Control By Cytoskeletal Interactions". *Proceedings of the National Academy of Sciences* 77 (5): 2537-2541. doi:10.1073/pnas.77.5.2537.

Gothoskar, A.V. 2004. "Resealed Erythrocytes: A Review", *Pharmaceutical Technology,* https://pdfs.semanticscholar.org/d0ae/ 6af93d98fb2bcdbc02c9617e39eb9affab73.pdf.

Gourley, D.R.H. 1957. "Human Erythrocyte Ghosts Prepared to Contain Various Metabolites*", Journal of Applied Physiology* 10:3, 511-518.

Grebowski, Jacek, Anita Krokosz, and Mieczyslaw Puchala. 2013. "Fullerenol C60(OH)36 Could Associate To Band 3 Protein Of Human Erythrocyte Membranes". *Biochimica Et Biophysica Acta (BBA) - Biomembranes* 1828 (9): 2007-2014. doi:10.1016/j.bbamem.2013. 05.009.

Gupta, Nilesh, Brijeshkumar Patel, and Fakhrul Ahsan. 2014. "Nano-Engineered Erythrocyte Ghosts as Inhalational Carriers for Delivery of Fasudil: Preparation and Characterization". *Pharmaceutical Research* 31 (6): 1553-1565. doi:10.1007/s11095-013-1261-7.

Hamidi, Mehrdad, Adbolhossein Zarrin, Mahshid Foroozesh, and Soliman Mohammadi-Samani. 2007a. "Applications of Carrier Erythrocytes in Delivery of Biopharmaceuticals". *Journal of Controlled Release* 118 (2): 145-160. doi:10.1016/j.jconrel.2006.06.032.

Hamidi, Mehrdad, Najmeh Zarei, Abdolhossein Zarrin, and Soleiman Mohammadi-Samani. 2007b. "Preparation and Validation of Carrier Human Erythrocytes Loaded By Bovine Serum Albumin as a Model Antigen/Protein". *Drug Delivery* 14 (5): 295-300. doi:10.1080/ 10717540701203000.

Hamidi, M., A.H. Zarrin, M. Foroozesh, N. Zarei, and S. Mohammadi-Samani. 2007c. "Preparation and In Vitro Evaluation of Carrier Erythrocytes for RES-Targeted Delivery of Interferon-Alpha 2B". *International Journal of Pharmaceutics* 341 (1-2): 125-133. doi:10.1016/j.ijpharm.2007.04.001.

Hamidi, Mehrdad, and Hosnieh Tajerzadeh. 2003. "Carrier Erythrocytes: An Overview". *Drug Delivery* 10 (1): 9-20. doi:10.1080/713840329.

Hamidi, Mehrdad, Hosnieh Tajerzadeh, Ahmad-Reza Dehpour, Mohammad-Reza Rouini and Shahram Ejtemaee-Mehr. 2001. "In vitro characterization of human intact erythrocytes loaded by enalaprilat". *Drug Delivery* 8:223-230.

Hamidi, Mehrdad, Pedram Rafiei, Amir Azadi, and Soliman Mohammadi-Samani. 2011. "Encapsulation of Valproate-Loaded Hydrogel Nanoparticles in Intact Human Erythrocytes: A Novel Nano-Cell Composite for Drug Delivery". *Journal of Pharmaceutical Sciences* 100 (5): 1702-1711. doi:10.1002/jps.22395.

Han, Xiao, Chao Wang, and Zhuang Liu. 2018. "Red Blood Cells as Smart Delivery Systems". *Bioconjugate Chemistry* 29 (4): 852-860. doi:10.1021/acs.bioconjchem.7b00758.

Harisa, Gamal El-din I., Mohammed F. Ibrahim, and Fars K. Alanazi. 2011. "Characterization of Human Erythrocytes as Potential Carrier for Pravastatin: An In Vitro Study". *International Journal of Medical Sciences* 8 (3): 222-230. doi:10.7150/ijms.8.222.

Harisa, Gamaleldin I., Mohamed F. Ibrahim, and Fars K. Alanazi. 2012. "Erythrocyte-Mediated Delivery Of Pravastatin: In Vitro Study of Effect of Hypotonic Lysis On Biochemical Parameters And Loading Efficiency". *Archives of Pharmacal Research* 35 (8): 1431-1439. doi:10.1007/s12272-012-0813-4.

Harisa, Gamaleldin I., Mohamed M. Badran, Saeed A. AlQahtani, Fars K. Alanazi, and Sabry M. Attia. 2016. "Pravastatin Chitosan Nanogels-Loaded Erythrocytes as a New Delivery Strategy for Targeting Liver Cancer". *Saudi Pharmaceutical Journal* 24 (1): 74-81. doi:10.1016/j.jsps.2015.03.024.

Harris, Faith M., Samantha K. Smith, and John D. Bell. 2001. "Physical Properties of Erythrocyte Ghosts That Determine Susceptibility to Secretory Phospholipase A2". *Journal of Biological Chemistry* 276 (25): 22722-22731. doi:10.1074/jbc.m010879200.

Harvey, John W. 2008. " The Erythrocyte: Physiology, Metabolism, and Biochemical Disorders". In *Clinical Biochemistry of Domestic Animals*, edited by Kaneko Jerry J., John W. Harvey, Michael L. Bruss, 173-238. New York: Academic Press.

Hinderling, Peter H. 1997 "Red blood cells: a neglected compartment in pharmacokinetics and pharmacodynamics". *Pharmacological Reviews* 49(3):279-295.

Hoffman, Joseph F. 1992. "On red blood cells, hemolysis and resealed ghosts". In: *The Use of Resealed Erythrocytes as Carriers and Bioreactors,* edited by Magnani Mauro, John DeLoach R, 1–15. New York: Plenum Publishing.

Holovati, Jelena L., Maria I.C. Gyongyossy-Issa, and Jason P. Acker. 2009. "Effects of Trehalose-Loaded Liposomes on Red Blood Cell Response to Freezing and Post-Thaw Membrane Quality". *Cryobiology* 58 (1): 75-83. doi:10.1016/j.cryobiol.2008.11.002.

Hsieh, Chen-Chan, Shih-Tsung Kang, Yee-Hsien Lin, Yi-Ju Ho, Chung-Hsin Wang, Chih-Kuang Yeh, and Chien-Wen Chang. 2015. "Biomimetic Acoustically-Responsive Vesicles for Theranostic Applications". *Theranostics* 5 (11): 1264-1274. doi:10.7150/thno.11848.

Hu, C.-M.J., L. Zhang, S. Aryal, C. Cheung, R.H. Fang, and L. Zhang. 2011. "Erythrocyte Membrane-Camouflaged Polymeric Nanoparticles as a Biomimetic Delivery Platform". *Proceedings of the National Academy of Sciences* 108 (27): 10980-10985. doi:10.1073/pnas.1106634108.

Hu, Che-Ming J., Ronnie H. Fang, Jonathan Copp, Brian T. Luk, and Liangfang Zhang. 2013. "A Biomimetic Nanosponge That Absorbs Pore-Forming Toxins". *Nature Nanotechnology* 8 (5): 336-340. doi:10.1038/nnano.2013.54.

Huang, Nai-Jia, Novalia Pishesha, Jean Mukherjee, Sicai Zhang, Rhogerry Deshycka, Valentino Sudaryo, Min Dong, Charles B. Shoemaker, and Harvey F. Lodish. 2017. "Genetically Engineered Red Cells Expressing Single Domain Camelid Antibodies Confer Long-Term Protection Against Botulinum Neurotoxin". *Nature Communications* 8 (1). doi:10.1038/s41467-017-00448-0.

Huang, Ping, Jing Zhao, Chiju Wei, Xiaohu Hou, Pingzhang Chen, Yan Tan, Cheng-Yi He, Zhiyong Wang, and Zhi-Ying Chen. 2016. "Erythrocyte Membrane Based Cationic Polymer-Mcdna Complexes as an Efficient Gene Delivery System". *Biomaterials Science* 5 (1): 120-127. doi:10.1039/c6bm00638h.

Ihler, G.M., R.H. Glew, and F.W. Schnure. 1973. "Enzyme Loading of Erythrocytes". *Proceedings of the National Academy of Sciences* 70 (9): 2663-2666. doi:10.1073/pnas.70.9.2663.

Ihler, Garret M. 1983. "Erythrocyte carriers", *Pharmacology & Therapeutics* 20, 151-169.

Jain, Nemi C. 1993. *Essentials of Veterinary Hematology*, Lea & Febiger Philadelphia.

Jain, Sanjay and Narenda K. Jain. 2003. "Engineered Nanoerythrocytes as a Novel Drug Delivery System." In *Erythrocyte Engineering for Drug Delivery and Targeting, Biotechnology Intelligence Unit 6*, edited by Mauro Magnani, 77-92. Landes Bioscience/Eurekah.com and Kluwer Academic/Plenum Publisher.

Jain, Sanjay and Narenda K. Jain. 1997. "Engineered erythrocytes as a drug delivery system". *Indian Journal of Pharmaceutical Sciences.* 59: 275-281.

Jain, S., S.K. Jain, V.K. Dixit.1995. "Erythrocytes based delivery of isoniazid: preparation and in-vitro characterization". *Indian Drugs* 32:471–476.

Johnstone, James E., Leslie A. MacLaren, Jay Doucet, and Vivian C. McAlister. 2004. "In Vitro Studies Regarding the Feasibility of Bovine Erythrocyte Xenotransfusion". *Xenotransplantation* 11 (1): 11-17. doi:10.1111/j.1399-3089.2004.00070.x.

Kabaso, Doron, Roie Shlomovit, Thorsten Auth, Virgilio L. Lew, Nir S. Gov.. 2011. "Cytoskeletal Reorganization of Red Blood Cell Shape: Curling of Free Edges and Malaria Merozoites". In: (ed.) Iglic A., *Advances in Planar Lipid Bilayers and Liposomes,* Volume 13, pp. 73-102.

Kim, Sang-Hee, Eun-Joong Kim, Joon-Hyuk Hou, Jung-Mogg Kim, Han-Gon Choi, Chang-Koo Shim, and Yu-Kyoung Oh. 2009. "Opsonized Erythrocyte Ghosts for Liver-Targeted Delivery of Antisense Oligodeoxynucleotides". *Biomaterials* 30 (5): 959-967. doi:10.1016/j.biomaterials.2008.10.031.

Kontos, Stephan, and Jeffrey A. Hubbell. 2010. "Improving Protein Pharmacokinetics by Engineering Erythrocyte Affinity". *Molecular Pharmaceutics* 7 (6): 2141-2147. doi:10.1021/mp1001697.

Kostić, Ivana T. 2015. *"Preserved erythrocyte membranes produced from slaughterhouse blood as systems for prolonged delivery of active substances"*. PhD diss., University of Belgrade.

Kostić, Ivana T., Katarina S. Bukara, Radoslava Pravilović, Vesna Lj. Ilić, Slavko B. Mojsilović, Smilja D. Marković, Branko M. Bugarski. 2015b. "Morphological characterization of erythrocyte membranes derived from bovine and porcine slaughterhouse blood as dexamethasone sodium phosphate carriers". *Paper presented at IV International congress "Engineering, Environment and Materials in Processing Industry" Jahorina*, Republic of Srpska, Bosnia and Herzegovina, I-33-E pp. 312-317, 04th-06th March.

Kostić, Ivana T., Katarina Bukara, Vesna Ilić, Branko Bugarski. 2013. "Effect of bovine blood storage in slaughterhouses on parameters relevant to hemoglobin isolation". Paper presented at International 57th Meat Industry Conference *"Meat and meat products–perspectives of sustainable production"*, Belgrade, Serbia, pp. 201-205, 10-12 June.

Kostić, Ivana T., Vesna Lj. Ilić, Katarina M. Bukara, Slavko B. Mojsilović, Zorka Ž. Đurić, Petra P. Draškovič, Branko M. Bugarski. 2015. "Flow cytometric determination of osmotic behaviour of animal erythrocytes toward their engineering for drug delivery". *Hemijska industrija* 69(1) 67-76. DOI: 10.2298/HEMIND140124021K.

Kostić, Ivana T., Vesna Lj. Ilić, Verica B. Đorđević, Katarina M. Bukara, Slavko B. Mojsilović, Viktor A. Nedović, Diana S. Bugarski, Đorđe N. Veljović, Danijela M. Mišić, and Branko M. Bugarski. 2014. "Erythrocyte Membranes from Slaughterhouse Blood as Potential Drug Vehicles: Isolation by Gradual Hypotonic Hemolysis and Biochemical and Morphological Characterization". *Colloids and Surfaces B: Biointerfaces* 122: 250-259. doi:10.1016/j.colsurfb.2014.06.043.

Kravtzoff, R., C. Ropars, M. Laguerre, J.P. Muh, and M. Chassaigne. 1990. "Erythrocytes as Carriers for L-Asparaginase. Methodological and Mouse In-Vivo Studies". *Journal of Pharmacy and Pharmacology* 42 (7): 473-476. doi:10.1111/j.2042-7158.1990.tb06598.x.

Kreft, Oliver, Radostina Georgieva, Hans Bäumler, Martin Steup, Bernd Müller-Röber, Gleb B. Sukhorukov, and Helmuth Möhwald. 2006. "Red Blood Cell Templated Polyelectrolyte Capsules: A Novel Vehicle for the Stable Encapsulation of DNA and Proteins". *Macromolecular Rapid Communications* 27 (6): 435-440. doi:10.1002/marc.200500777.

Kuo, Yuan-Chia, Hsuan-Chen Wu, Dao Hoang, William E. Bentley, Warren D. D'Souza, and Srinivasa R. Raghavan. 2016. "Colloidal Properties of Nanoerythrosomes Derived From Bovine Red Blood Cells". *Langmuir* 32 (1): 171-179. doi:10.1021/acs.langmuir.5b03014.

Lautenschläger, Christian, Carsten Schmidt, Dagmar Fischer, and Andreas Stallmach. 2014. "Drug Delivery Strategies in the Therapy of Inflammatory Bowel Disease". *Advanced Drug Delivery Reviews* 71: 58-76. doi:10.1016/j.addr.2013.10.001.

Lejeune, A., M. Moorjani, C. Gicquaud, J. Lacroix, P. Poyet, R. Gaudreault. 1994. "Nanoerythrosome, a new derivative of erythrocyte ghost: preparation and antineoplastic potential as drug carrier for daunorubicin". *Anticancer Research* 14 (3A):915-919.

"L-Asparaginase Encapsulated In Red Blood Cells (Eryaspase) For Treatment of Adult Patients with ALL or LBL - Full Text View - Clinicaltrials.Gov". 2019. *Clinicaltrials.Gov*. https://clinicaltrials.gov/ct2/show/NCT01910428?term=L-asparaginase&rank=1.

Lieber, Michael R., and Theodore L. Steck. 1989. "Hemolytic holes in human erythrocyte membrane ghosts." *Methods in Enzymology* 173:356–367. https://doi.org/10.1016/S0076-6879(89)73023-8.

Lizano, Carmen, M. Teresa Pérez, and Montserrat Pinilla. 2001. "Mouse Erythrocytes as Carriers for Coencapsulated Alcohol and Aldehyde Dehydrogenase Obtained By Electroporation". *Life Sciences* 68 (17): 2001-2016. doi:10.1016/s0024-3205(01)00991-2.

Lodish, Harvey, Arnold Berk, S. Lawrence Zipursky, Paul Matsudaira, David Baltimore, and James Darnell. Molecular Cell Biology, 4th edition, New York: W.H. Freeman; 2000. ISBN-10: 0-7167-3136-3.

Section 5.3, *Biomembranes: Structural Organization and Basic Functions*. Available from: https://www.ncbi.nlm.nih.gov/books/NBK21583/

Luk, Brian T., and Liangfang Zhang. 2015. "Cell Membrane-Camouflaged Nanoparticles for Drug Delivery". *Journal of Controlled Release* 220: 600-607. doi:10.1016/j.jconrel.2015.07.019.

Luk, Brian. 2016. *"Cell Membrane-Cloaked Nanoparticles for Targeted Therapeutics"*, PhD diss., UC San Diego.

Luna, E.J., and A.L. Hitt. 1992. "Cytoskeleton--plasma membrane interactions", *Science* 258(5084): 955-964, doi: 10.1126/science.1439807.

Lux, Samuel E. 2016. "Anatomy of the Red Cell Membrane Skeleton: Unanswered Questions". *Blood* 127 (2): 187-199. doi:10.1182/blood-2014-12-512772.

Lynch, Sarah A., Anne Maria Mullen, Eileen E. O'Neill, and Carlos Álvarez García. 2017. "Harnessing the Potential of Blood Proteins As Functional Ingredients: A Review of the State of the Art in Blood Processing". *Comprehensive Reviews in Food Science and Food Safety* 16 (2): 330-344. doi:10.1111/1541-4337.12254.

Magnani, M., L. Rossi, G. Brandi, G.F. Schiavano, M. Montroni, and G. Piedimonte. 1992. "Targeting Antiretroviral Nucleoside Analogues in Phosphorylated Form to Macrophages: In Vitro and In Vivo Studies.". *Proceedings of the National Academy of Sciences* 89 (14): 6477-6481. doi:10.1073/pnas.89.14.6477.

Magnani, Mauro, Luigia Rossi, Marcello D'Ascenzo, Ivo Panzani, Leonardo Bigi, Andrea Zanella. 1998. "Erythrocyte engineering for drug delivery and targeting". *Biotechnology and Applied Biochemistry* 28: 1-6.

Mambrini, Giovanni, Marco Mandolini, Luigia Rossi, Francesca Pierigè, Giovanni Capogrossi, Patricia Salvati, Sonja Serafini, Luca Benatti, and Mauro Magnani. 2017. "Ex Vivo Encapsulation of Dexamethasone Sodium Phosphate Into Human Autologous Erythrocytes Using Fully Automated Biomedical Equipment".

International Journal of Pharmaceutics 517 (1-2): 175-184. doi:10.1016/j.ijpharm.2016.12.011.

Mansouri, Sania, Yahye Merhi, Françoise M. Winnik, and Maryam Tabrizian. 2011. "Investigation of Layer-By-Layer Assembly of Polyelectrolytes on Fully Functional Human Red Blood Cells in Suspension for Attenuated Immune Response". *Biomacromolecules* 12 (3): 585-592. doi:10.1021/bm101200c.

Martín-Sabroso, Cristina, Daniel Filipe Tavares-Fernandes, Juan Ignacio Espada-García, and Ana Isabel Torres-Suárez. 2013. "Validation Protocol of Analytical Procedures for Quantification of Drugs in Polymeric Systems for Parenteral Administration: Dexamethasone Phosphate Disodium Microparticles". *International Journal of Pharmaceutics* 458 (1): 188-196. doi:10.1016/j.ijpharm.2013.09.026.

Matsuzawa, Toshiaki, and Yasushi Ikarashi. 1979. "Haemolysis of Various Mammalian Erythrocytes in Sodium Chloride, Glucose and Phosphate-Buffer Solutions". *Laboratory Animals* 13 (4): 329-331. doi:10.1258/002367779780943297.

Millán, Carmen Gutiérrez, María Luisa Sayalero Marinero, Aránzazu Zarzuelo Castañeda, and José M. Lanao. 2004a. "Drug, Enzyme and Peptide Delivery Using Erythrocytes As Carriers". *Journal of Controlled Release* 95 (1): 27-49. doi:10.1016/j.jconrel.2003.11.018.

Millán, Carmen G., Aránzazu Zarzuelo Castañeda, María Luisa Sayalero Marinero, and José M. Lanao. 2004b. "Factors Associated With The Performance Of Carrier Erythrocytes Obtained By Hypotonic Dialysis". *Blood Cells, Molecules, and Diseases* 33 (2): 132-140. doi:10.1016/j.bcmd.2004.06.004.

Millán, Carmen G., Bridget E. Bax, Aránzazu Zarzuelo Castañeda, María Luisa Sayalero Marinero, and José M. Lanao. 2008. "In Vitro Studies of Amikacin-Loaded Human Carrier Erythrocytes". *Translational Research* 152 (2): 59-66. doi:10.1016/j.trsl.2008.05.008.

Millán, Carmen G., Diana Galván Bravo, and José M. Lanao. 2017. "New Erythrocyte-Related Delivery Systems for Biomedical Applications". *Journal of Drug Delivery Science and Technology* 42: 38-48. doi:10.1016/j.jddst.2017.03.019.

Mishra, P.R., and N.K. Jain. 2003. "Folate Conjugated Doxorubicin-Loaded Membrane Vesicles For Improved Cancer Therapy". *Drug Delivery* 10 (4): 277-282. doi:10.1080/714044320.

Montes, L.-Ruth, David J. López, Jesús Sot, Luis A. Bagatolli, Martin J. Stonehouse, Michael L. Vasil, Bill X. Wu, Yusuf A. Hannun, Félix M. Goñi, and Alicia Alonso. 2008. "Ceramide-Enriched Membrane Domains in Red Blood Cells and the Mechanism of Sphingomyelinase-Induced Hot−Cold Hemolysis". *Biochemistry* 47 (43): 11222-11230. doi:10.1021/bi801139z.

Moorjani, M., A. Lejeune, C. Gicquaud, J. Lacroix, P. Poyet, R.C. Gaudreault. 1996. "Nanoerythrosomes, a new derivative of erythrocyte ghost II: identification of the mechanism of action". *Anticancer Research* 16:2831-2836.

Mota-Rojas, D., M. Becerril-Herrera, P. Roldan-Santiago, M. Alonso-Spilsbury, S. Flores-Peinado, R. Ramírez-Necoechea, and J.A. Ramírez-Telles et al. 2012. "Effects of Long Distance Transportation and CO2 Stunning on Critical Blood Values in Pigs". *Meat Science* 90 (4): 893-898. doi:10.1016/j.meatsci.2011.11.027.

Murciano, Juan-Carlos, Sandra Medinilla, Donald Eslin, Elena Atochina, Douglas B. Cines, and Vladimir R. Muzykantov. 2003. "Prophylactic Fibrinolysis through Selective Dissolution of Nascent Clots by tPA-Carrying Erythrocytes". *Nature Biotechnology* 21 (8): 891-896. doi:10.1038/nbt846.

Muzykantov, Vladimir R. 2010. "Drug Delivery by Red Blood Cells: Vascular Carriers Designed By Mother Nature". *Expert Opinion on Drug Delivery* 7 (4): 403-427. doi:10.1517/17425241003610633.

Nash, G.B., and H.J. Meiselman. 1983. "Red Cell and Ghost Viscoelasticity. Effects of Hemoglobin Concentration and In Vivo Aging". *Biophysical Journal* 43 (1): 63-73. doi:10.1016/s0006-3495(83)84324-0.

"*Open-Label, Long-Term, Extension Treatment Using Intra-Erythrocyte Dexamethasone Sodium Phosphate in Patients with Ataxia Telangiectasia Who Participated in the IEDAT-02-2015 Study - Full Text View - Clinicaltrials.Gov*". 2019. Clinicaltrials.Gov. https://

clinicaltrials.gov/ct2/show/NCT03563053?term=EryDex+System&rank=3.

Pajic-Lijakovic, Ivana, and Milan Milivojevic. 2014. "Modeling Analysis of the Lipid Bilayer–Cytoskeleton Coupling In Erythrocyte Membrane". *Biomechanics and Modeling in Mechanobiology* 13 (5): 1097-1104. doi:10.1007/s10237-014-0559-7.

Pajic-Lijakovic, Ivana, and Milan Milivojevic. 2017. "Viscoelasticity of Multicellular Surfaces". *Journal of Biomechanics* 60: 1-8. doi:10.1016/j.jbiomech.2017.06.035.

Pajic-Lijakovic, Ivana, Vesna Ilic, Branko Bugarski, and Milenko Plavsic. 2010. "Rearrangement of Erythrocyte Band 3 Molecules and Reversible Formation of Osmotic Holes under Hypotonic Conditions". *European Biophysics Journal with Biophysics Letters,* 39 (5): 789-800. doi: 10.1007/s00249-009-0554-6.

Pajic-Lijakovic, Ivana. 2015a. "Erythrocytes under osmotic stress–modeling considerations". *Progress in Biophysics and Molecular Biology 117*(1):113-124.

Pajic-Lijakovic, Ivana. 2015b. "Role of Band 3 in Erythrocyte Membrane Structural Changes under Thermal Fluctuations-Modeling Considerations". *Journal of Bioenergetics and Biomembranes* 47(6):507-518.

Patel P.D., N. Dand, R.S. Hirlekar, and V.J. Kadam 2008. "Drug Loaded Erythrocytes: As Novel Drug Delivery System", *Current Pharmaceutical Design,* 14: 63-70.

Piagnerelli, M., K. Zouaoui Boudjeltia, D. Brohee, A. Vereerstraeten, P. Piro, J-L. Vincent, and M. Vanhaeverbeek. 2007. "Assessment of Erythrocyte Shape by Flow Cytometry Techniques". *Journal of Clinical Pathology* 60 (5): 549-554. doi:10.1136/jcp.2006.037523.

Piao, Ji-Gang, Limin Wang, Feng Gao, Ye-Zi You, Yujie Xiong, and Lihua Yang. 2014. "Erythrocyte Membrane Is An Alternative Coating To Polyethylene Glycol For Prolonging The Circulation Lifetime Of Gold Nanocages For Photothermal Therapy". *ACS Nano* 8 (10): 10414-10425. doi:10.1021/nn503779d.

Pierigè, Francesca, Noemi Bigini, Luigia Rossi, and Mauro Magnani. 2017. "Reengineering Red Blood Cells for Cellular Therapeutics and Diagnostics". *Wiley Interdisciplinary Reviews: Nanomedicine And Nanobiotechnology* 9 (5): e1454. doi:10.1002/wnan.1454.

Pishesha, Novalia, Angelina M. Bilate, Marsha C. Wibowo, Nai-Jia Huang, Zeyang Li, Rhogerry Dhesycka, and Djenet Bousbaine et al. 2017. "Engineered Erythrocytes Covalently Linked To Antigenic Peptides Can Protect Against Autoimmune Disease". *Proceedings of the National Academy of Sciences* 114 (12): 3157-3162. doi:10.1073/pnas.1701746114.

Podlubny, Igor. 1999. *Fractional differential equations, mathematics in science and engineering,* Vol 198. London, Academic Press, p 78.

Pouliot, Roxane, Audrey Saint-Laurent, Camille Chypre, Ritchie Audet, Isabelle Vitté-Mony, René C. Gaudreault, Michèle Auger. 2002. "Spectroscopic characterization of nanoErythrosomes in the absence and presence of conjugated polyethyleneglycols: an FTIR and 31P-NMR study". *Biochimica et Biophysica Acta* 1564: 317– 324.

Pravilovic, Radoslava, Slavko Mojsilovic, Ivana Kostic, Vesna Ilic, Diana Bugarski, Verica Djordjevic, and Branko Bugarski. 2012. "Optimization of Gradual Hemolysis for Isolation of Hemoglobin from Bovine Erythrocytes". *Hemijska industrija* 66 (4): 519-529. doi:10.2298/hemind111122008s.

Pribush, Alexander, Dan Meyerstein, and Naomi Meyerstein. 2002. "Kinetics of Erythrocyte Swelling and Membrane Hole Formation in Hypotonic Media". *Biochimica et Biophysica Acta (BBA) - Biomembranes* 1558 (2): 119-132. doi: 10.1016/s0005-2736(01)00418-7.

Rivas, Isabel Patricia, María Esther Gil-Alegre, and Ana Isabel Torres-Suárez. 2006. "Development and Validation of A Fast High-Performance Liquid Chromatography Method for the Determination of Microencapsulated Pyrethroid Pesticides". *Analytica Chimica Acta* 557 (1-2): 245-251. doi:10.1016/j.aca.2005.10.042.

Rossi, Luigia, Sonja Serafini, Loredana Cappellacci, Emanuela Balestra, Giorgio Brandi, Giuditta F. Schiavano, Palmarisa Franchetti, Mario

Grifantini, Carlo-Federico Perno, Mauro Magnani. 2001a. "Erythrocyte-Mediated Delivery of a New Homodinucleotide Active Against Human Immunodeficiency Virus And Herpes Simplex Virus". *Journal of Antimicrobial Chemotherapy* 47 (6): 819-827. doi:10.1093/jac/47.6.819.

Rossi, Luigia, Sonja Serafini, Luigi Cenerini, Francesco Picardi, Leonardo Bigi, Ivo Panzani, and Mauro Magnani. 2001b. "Erythrocyte-Mediated Delivery of Dexamethasone in Patients with Chronic Obstructive Pulmonary Disease". *Biotechnology and Applied Biochemistry* 33 (2): 85. doi:10.1042/ba20000087.

Rossi, Luigia, Francesca Pierigè, Antonella Antonelli, Noemi Bigini, Claudia Gabucci, Enrico Peiretti, and Mauro Magnani. 2016. "Engineering Erythrocytes for the Modulation of Drugs' and Contrasting Agents' Pharmacokinetics and Biodistribution". *Advanced Drug Delivery Reviews* 106: 73-87. doi:10.1016/j.addr.2016.05.008.

Rossi, Luigia, Massimo Castro, Francesco D'Orio, Gianluca Damonte, Sonja Serafini, Leonardo Bigi, and Ivo Panzani et al. 2004. "Low Doses Of Dexamethasone Constantly Delivered By Autologous Erythrocytes Slow The Progression Of Lung Disease In Cystic Fibrosis Patients". *Blood Cells, Molecules and Diseases* 33 (1): 57-63. doi:10.1016/j.bcmd.2004.04.004.

Sato, Yukio, Hiroshi Yamakose, and Yasuo Suzuki. 1993. "Mechanism of Hypotonic Hemolysis of Human Erythrocytes." *Biological & Pharmaceutical Bulletin* 16 (5): 506-512. doi:10.1248/bpb.16.506.

Schwoch, G. and H. Passow. 1973 "Preparation and properties of human erythrocyte ghosts". *Molecular and Cellular Biochemistry* 2:197–218. https://doi.org/10.1007/BF01795474.

Shaillender, Mutukumaraswamy, Rongcong Luo, Subbu S. Venkatraman, and Björn Neu. 2011. "Layer-By-Layer Microcapsules Templated on Erythrocyte Ghost Carriers". *International Journal of Pharmaceutics* 415 (1-2): 211-217. doi:10.1016/j.ijpharm.2011.06.011.

Shi, J., L. Kundrat, N. Pishesha, A. Bilate, C. Theile, T. Maruyama, S.K. Dougan, H.L. Ploegh, and H.F. Lodish. 2014. "Engineered Red Blood Cells As Carriers For Systemic Delivery of a Wide Array of Functional

Probes". *Proceedings of the National Academy of Sciences* 111 (28): 10131-10136. doi:10.1073/pnas.1409861111.

Shlomovitz, R., and N.S. Gov. 2008. "Exciting Cytoskeleton-Membrane Waves". *Physical Review E* 78 (4). doi:10.1103/physreve.78.041911.

Staedtke, V., M. Brähler, A. Müller, R. Georgieva, S. Bauer, N. Sternberg, and A. Voigt et al. 2010. "In Vitro Inhibition of Fungal Activity by Macrophage-Mediated Sequestration and Release of Encapsulated Amphotericin B Nanosupension in Red Blood Cells". *Small* 6 (1): 96-103. doi:10.1002/smll.200900919.

Sternberg, Nadine, Radostina Georgieva, Karolin Duft, and Hans Bäumler. 2011. "Surface-Modified Loaded Human Red Blood Cells for Targeting and Delivery of Drugs". *Journal of Microencapsulation* 29 (1): 9-20. doi:10.3109/02652048.2011.629741.

Stojanović, Radoslava, Vesna Ilić, Verica Manojlović, Diana Bugarski, Marija Dević, and Branko Bugarski. 2012. "Isolation of Hemoglobin from Bovine Erythrocytes by Controlled Hemolysis in the Membrane Bioreactor". *Applied Biochemistry and Biotechnology* 166 (6): 1491-1506. doi:10.1007/s12010-012-9543-9.

Sun, M., N. Northup, F. Marga, T. Huber, F.J. Byfield, I. Levitan, and G. Forgacs. 2007. "The Effect of Cellular Cholesterol on Membrane-Cytoskeleton Adhesion". *Journal of Cell Science* 120 (13): 2223-2231. doi:10.1242/jcs.001370.

Tajerzadeh, Hosnieh, and Mehrdad Hamidi. 2000. "Evaluation of Hypotonic -ling Method for Encapsulation of Enalaprilat in Intact Human Erythrocytes". *Drug Development and Industrial Pharmacy* 26 (12): 1247-1257. doi:10.1081/ddc-100102306.

Talwar, N., and N.K. Jaind. 1992. "Erythrocyte Based Delivery System of Primaquine: *In Vitro* characterization". *Journal of Microencapsulation* 9 (3): 357-364. doi:10.3109/02652049209021250.

van den Bos, Cor, Francis C.J.M. van Gils, Rolf W. Bartstra, and Gerard Wagemaker. 1992. "Flow Cytometric Analysis of Peripheral Blood Erythrocyte Chimerism in A-Thalassemic Mice". *Cytometry* 13 (6): 659-662. doi:10.1002/cyto.990130616.

Villa, Carlos H., Aaron C. Anselmo, Samir Mitragotri, and Vladimir Muzykantov. 2016. "Red Blood Cells: Supercarriers for Drugs, Biologicals, and Nanoparticles and Inspiration for Advanced Delivery Systems". *Advanced Drug Delivery Reviews* 106: 88-103. doi:10.1016/j.addr.2016.02.007.

Villa, Carlos H., Douglas B. Cines, Don L. Siegel, and Vladimir Muzykantov. 2017. "Erythrocytes as Carriers for Drug Delivery in Blood Transfusion and Beyond". *Transfusion Medicine Reviews* 31 (1): 26-35. doi:10.1016/j.tmrv.2016.08.004.

Villa, Carlos H., Jerard Seghatchian, and Vladimir Muzykantov. 2016. "Drug Delivery by Erythrocytes: "Primum Non Nocere"". *Transfusion and Apheresis Science* 55 (3): 275-280. doi:10.1016/j.transci.2016.10.017.

Vitvitsky, V.M., E.V. Frolova, M.V. Martinov, S.V. Komarova, and F.I. Ataullakhanov. 2000. "Anion Permeability and Erythrocyte Swelling". *Bioelectrochemistry* 52 (2): 169-177. doi:10.1016/s0302-4598(00)00099-4.

Wali, Ramesh K., Stuart Jaffe, Dinesh Kumar, Nino Sorgente, and Vijay K. Kalra. 1987. "Increased Adherence of Oxidant-Treated Human and Bovine Erythrocytes to Cultured Endothelial Cells". *Journal of Cellular Physiology* 133 (1): 25-36. doi:10.1002/jcp.1041330104.

Webb, M.S., T.O. Harasym, D. Masin, M.B. Bally, and L.D. Mayer. 1995. "Sphingomyelin-Cholesterol Liposomes Significantly Enhance the Pharmacokinetic and Therapeutic Properties of Vincristine in Murine and Human Tumour Models". *British Journal of Cancer* 72 (4): 896-904. doi:10.1038/bjc.1995.430.

Yoo, Jin-Wook, Darrell J. Irvine, Dennis E. Discher, and Samir Mitragotri. 2011. "Bio-Inspired, Bioengineered and Biomimetic Drug Delivery Carriers". *Nature Reviews Drug Discovery* 10 (7): 521-535. doi:10.1038/nrd3499.

Yousefpour, Parisa, and Ashutosh Chilkoti. 2014. "Co-Opting Biology to Deliver Drugs". *Biotechnology And Bioengineering* 111 (9): 1699-1716. doi:10.1002/bit.25307.

Zade-Oppen, A.M.M. 1998. "Repetitive Cell 'Jumps' During Hypotonic Lysis of Erythrocytes Observed With a Simple Flow Chamber". *Journal of Microscopy* 192 (1): 54-62. doi:10.1046/j.1365-2818.1998.00402.x.

Zaitsev, Sergei, Kristina Danielyan, Juan-Carlos Murciano, Kumkum Ganguly, Tatiana Krasik, Ronald P. Taylor, Steven Pincus, Steven Jones, Douglas B. Cines, and Vladimir R. Muzykantov. 2006. "Human Complement Receptor Type 1-Directed Loading of Tissue Plasminogen Activator on Circulating Erythrocytes For Prophylactic Fibrinolysis". *Blood* 108 (6): 1895-1902. doi:10.1182/blood-2005-11-012336.

Zhang, Haijun. 2016. "Erythrocytes in Nanomedicine: An Optimal Blend of Natural and Synthetic Materials". *Biomaterial Sciences* 4 (7): 1024-1031. doi:10.1039/c6bm00072j.

BIOGRAPHICAL SKETCH

Ivana T. Drvenica (née Kostić)

Affiliation: Institute for Medical Research, University of Belgrade

Education:
2010-2015 Ph.D., University of Belgrade, Serbia, Faculty of Technology and Metallurgy PhD thesis: "Preserved erythrocyte membranes produced from slaughterhouse blood as systems for prolonged delivery of active substances" (Module: Biochemical engineering and biotechnology)
2003-2009 M.Sc. Pharm., University of Belgrade, Serbia, Faculty of Pharmacy

Research and Professional Experience:
2011-present: Research team member on national project Reg. no. III 46010 funded by Ministry of Education, Science and

Technological Development of Republic of Serbia. "Novel encapsulation and enzyme technologies for designing of new biocatalyst and biologically active compounds targeting enhancement of food quality, safety and competitiveness."

2016-2017: Project coordinator of bilateral technical and scientific cooperation project between Republic of Serbia and Republic of Croatia: "Enhancement of the stability and bioavailability of phytochemicals by using different delivery systems and mathematical modeling of an *in vitro* gastrointestinal simulation."

2015-2018: MC substitute in COST action TD1306 "New Frontiers of Peer Review (PEERE)."

2014: MC substitute in COST action FA1001 "The application of innovative fundamental food-structure-property relationships to the design of foods for health, wellness and pleasure."

2012-2013: Research team member on technical and scientific cooperation project between Republic of Serbia and Republic of Portugal: "Stabilization of natural bioactive compounds: study of encapsulation techniques and release study."

2012-2013: Research team member on technical and scientific cooperation project between Republic of Serbia and Republic of Slovenia: "Hemoglobin from renewable source as a starting material for a heme-iron product for prevention and therapy of anemia in domestic animals: optimization of process of isolation and purification of hemoglobin."

2011-2012: Research team member on technical and scientific cooperation project between Republic of Serbia and Republic of Slovenia: "New micro-carrier systems for controlled drug delivery."

Professional Appointments:

2017-present:
Institute for Medical Research, University of Belgrade, Serbia
Assistant Professor of Research (Full time)
Laboratory for Immunology

2018-present:
Association of Chemical Engineers of Serbia
Secretary General (Part time)
2012-present:
Journal *Hemijska industrija*
(ISSN 0367-598X, http://www.ache.org.rs/HI/)
Assistant to Editor-in-Chief (Part time)
2012-2017:
Innovation center of Faculty of Technology and Metallurgy
Research Assistant (Full time)
Laboratory for Pharmaceutical Engineering

Publications from the Last 3 Years:
Drvenica, Ivana T., Katarina M. Bukara, Vesna Lj. Ilić, Danijela M. Mišić, Borislav Z. Vasić, Radoš B. Gajić, Verica B. Đorđević, Đorđe N. Veljović, Aleksandar Belić, and Branko M. Bugarski. 2016. "Biomembranes from Slaughterhouse Blood Erythrocytes as Prolonged Release Systems for Dexamethasone Sodium Phosphate". *Biotechnology Progress* 32 (4): 1046-1055. doi:10.1002/btpr.2304.

Bukara, Katarina, Ivana Drvenica, Vesna Ilić, Ana Stančić, Danijela Mišić, Borislav Vasić, Radoš Gajić, Dušan Vučetić, Filip Kiekens, and Branko Bugarski. 2016. "Comparative Studies on Osmosis Based Encapsulation of Sodium Diclofenac in Porcine and Outdated Human Erythrocyte Ghosts". *Journal of Biotechnology* 240: 14-22. doi:10.1016/j.jbiotec.2016.10.017.

Bukara, Katarina, Svetlana Jovanić, Ivana T. Drvenica, Ana Stančić, Vesna Ilić, Mihailo D. Rabasović, Dejan Pantelić, Branislav Jelenković, Branko Bugarski, Aleksandar Krmpot. 2017. "Mapping of hemoglobin in erythrocytes and erythrocyte ghosts using two photon excitation fluorescence microscopy". *Journal of Biomedical Optics* 22(2): 026003 http://dx.doi.org/10.1117/1.JBO.22.2.026003.

Trivanović, Drenka, Ivana Drvenica, Tamara Kukolj, Hristina Obradović, Ivana Okić Djordjević, Slavko Mojsilović, Jelena Krstić, Branko Bugarski, Aleksandra Jauković, Diana Bugarski. 2018.

"Adipoinductive Effect of Extracellular Matrix Involves Cytoskeleton Changes and SIRT1 Activity in Adipose Tissue Stem/Stromal Cells". *Artificial Cells, Nanomedicine, and Biotechnology,* https://doi.org/10.1080/21691401.2018.1494183.

Dobričić, Vladimir*, Ivana Drvenica*, Ana Stančić, Marija Mihailović, Olivera Čudina, Diana Bugarski, and Vesna Ilić. 2018. "Investigation Of Metabolic Properties And Effects Of 17B-Carboxamide Glucocorticoids On Human Peripheral Blood Leukocytes". *Archiv Der Pharmazie* 351 (5): 1700371. doi:10.1002/ardp.201700371. *authors equally contributed.

In: Erythrocytes
Editor: Katy Jorissen

ISBN: 978-1-53615-914-1
© 2019 Nova Science Publishers, Inc.

Chapter 4

ELECTROCHEMICAL PROPERTIES OF ERYTHROCYTES AS A REFLECTION OF THEIR MORPHOLOGY AND INTERACTION WITH FOREIGN ELECTRICALLY CONDUCTIVE MATERIALS

Mark M. Goldin[1],*, I. V. Goroncharovskaya[2], A. K. Evseev[2], A. K. Shabanov[2], Michael M. Goldin[1] and S. S. Petrikov[2]

[1]Glen Oaks Community College, Centreville, MI, US
[2]N. V. Sklifosovsky Research Institute of Emergency Medicine, Moscow, Russia

ABSTRACT

The electrochemical properties of blood cells play an important role in maintaining cell stability and biological function, and they are the deciding factor in the interaction of blood cells with both foreign materials and bodily tissues. Therefore, it is very important to investigate

---

* Corresponding Author's E-mail: markmgold@gmail.com

the electrochemical behavior of blood cells. The application of an electrochemical approach to rationalizing blood cell behavior in contact with foreign electrical conductors opens up opportunities for the development of novel analytical and diagnostic methods. The present work investigated the electrochemical behavior of erythrocytes (red blood cells) at platinum, carbonaceous, and optically transparent electrodes via polarization and coulometric measurements. Electrochemical activity of red blood cells was shown in both cathodic and anodic potential ranges of the above electrodes. The interaction of blood cells with the charged electrode surface was accompanied by electron transfer and changes in the morphology of cell membranes. The directionality of electron transfer and concomitant cell morphology changes were found to be dependent on the electrode potential. The order of magnitude of the quantity of electrons transferred between erythrocytes and electrodes was determined, and potential ranges showing indifference of the electrode toward red blood cells were identified. These results can be used to develop a method for evaluating the condition of normal and pathological erythrocytes, as well as to test novel materials for hemocompatibility.

INTRODUCTION

The electrochemical nature of the majority of important physiological processes has long been established. Therefore, applying electrochemical concepts, models and methods in biological systems provides ever-expanding insights into the homeostasis mechanisms that maintain self-regulation of the systems in the human body in response to external changes. Cellular-level homeostasis is a crucial aspect of self-regulation; via a number of equilibrium processes, it maintains cell health in the body's tissues and organs.

These considerations underlie the steady interest in electrochemical properties of blood cells in the literature that has not waned over many years. As far back as the 1930s, Abramson investigated the influence of electrochemical properties of blood cells on their behavior in electrolyte solutions using electrophoresis, and he also described biological and medical aspects of electrokinetic phenomena (Abramson 1934; Abramson et al. 1939). This method determined not only the magnitude and sign of the surface charges on cell membranes, but also their chemical composition. Other significant contributions in this realm were made by Ponder (Abramson 1939; Furchgott and Ponder 1941), Seaman (Seaman 1973; Seaman and Vassar 1966) and Kharamonenko (Kharamonenko and Rakityanskaya 1974).

Blood cell interaction with foreign materials was hypothesized to be electrochemical in nature because of the presence of excess negative charge on surface of cell membrane, as well as the existence of an electric double layer around the cell and the existence of charge on the foreign material surface. The use of an electrical conductor (activated carbon) as the foreign material serving as one of the electrodes in an electrochemical system comprising blood and carbon provided direct evidence of electrochemical interactions, which led to the development of an electrochemical model of blood cell interaction with foreign materials (Goldin et al. 2006).

Similarly, when non-conductive foreign materials are involved, electrostatic interaction with blood cells is observed. Indeed, the effect of electrostatic surface charge density of non-conductive Teflon on the degree of platelet lysis was shown in by Chepurov and Mertsalova, while the effect of charge density of non-metallic materials on their thrombogenicity (ability to cause blood clotting) was investigated by Sawyer (Chepurov and Mertsalova 1978).

Indeed, Sawyer's work made the most significant contribution to the understanding of blood cell interactions with vascular walls and foreign materials (Sawyer et al. 1974; Sawyer 1983). It was also the first to operationalize the electrochemical properties of foreign materials as a hemocompatibility selection criterion for implant materials. Measurements of potential on the platinum electrode implanted into a blood vessel wall led Sawyer to an important conclusion about the charge on the normal inner layer of vascular wall (*tunica intima*), *viz.*, that it is negatively charged with respect to the outer layer (*tunica adventitia*). Importantly, Sawyer's work showed that vascular injury led to a reversal in the sign of the *intima* charge from negative to positive (Sawyer and Pate 1953). Moreover, implanting a positively charged electrode into the *tunica adventitia* initiated local thrombus (clot) formation on the corresponding surface of the *intima*, while implanting a negatively charged platinum electrode into the *adventitia* did not cause such thrombus formation (Sawyer 1983).

Thus, the sign of the foreign material's charge was shown to exert major influence on the locally occurring blood clotting process. When different materials (including metals) were used to model an artificial vascular wall in the absence of external polarization, bringing these materials in contact with blood resulted in thrombus formation on the metals whose measured open-circuit potential (OCP) values were positive (Cu, Ni, Au, Pt) and did not result in clotting on metals with negative OCP values (Mg, Al, Cd) (Srinivasan and Sawyer 1970). It was also shown that non-thrombogenic properties can be imparted to a metal surface by changing the potential of the metal (Sawyer 1984). This is in agreement with the results obtained on activated carbons in contact with blood (Goldin et al. 1980; Luzhnikov et al. 1980).

A further investigation of the mechanism of foreign material-related thrombogenesis was performed on the above metals polarized to positive potentials (Sawyer et al. 1967). In these experiments, changes to blood cells occurred when the metal surface exceeded a certain "critical" positive potential value, and the observed changes were rationalized as a decrease in the mutual repulsion of blood cells occurring subsequent to a reduction in the negative charge density of the cell membranes. The process of deposition/removal of blood cells on the surface of platinum and gold was reversible at potentials between 0.51 to 0.55 V against the silver/silver chloride for erythrocytes and leukocytes and between 0.60 V to 0.65 V for platelets (Sawyer et al. 1965).

Based on this evidence, an electrochemical mechanism of interactions between blood cells and metals can be rationalized (Sawyer et al. 1964), with increased thrombogenicity of positively charged metal surfaces and, contrariwise, reduced thrombogenicity of negatively charged metal surfaces that are able to transfer electrons (and thereby impart negative charge) to the cell membranes. It should, of course, be noted that the electrochemical interactions between blood cells and metal surfaces cannot serve as a complete model of the thrombogenesis process (clot formation) without additional consideration of the electrochemical influences on the homeostatic processes occurring when blood cells come into contact with foreign surfaces or when a blood vessel is injured.

As shown by Michelson (2012), coagulation involves both a cellular (platelet) and a protein (coagulation factor) component. When vascular wall injury occurs, the underlying collagen directly binds the platelets circulating in the bloodstream. Substances released from both platelets and the vascular wall endothelium strengthen the adhesion and trigger a signaling cascade that activates platelets in a chain reaction, aggregating platelets via both mutual adhesion and adhesion to the damaged tissue to provide a platelet "plug." Signaling substances released by activated platelets also result in a coagulation cascade at the injury site involving fibrin formation from fibrinogen in the blood to cross-link the platelet plug, stabilizing it in the form of a fibrin clot. Absent injury and resulting platelet activation that triggers this cascade, the clotting proteins in the blood are present in an inactive form. The coagulation cascade is maintained in a prothrombotic state until it is down-regulated by the anticoagulant pathways.

It is also important that vessel embolization can be controlled by varying the value of the electrochemical potential (i.e., the charge density) of the foreign material surface (Evseev et al. 2014). Based on the "forced" thrombus formation effect, an intravascular medical treatment utilizing electrochemically controlled coagulation was developed, and it is utilized for the treatment of acute hemorrhages and aneurysms in vascular surgery (Evseev et al. 2014; Ji, Guglielmi and Chen 1997).

Electrochemical representations have been successfully used to investigate the processes of transmembrane electron transport in bacterial cells, which possess certain structural and functional similarities to blood cells. A number of investigations (Delaney et al. 1984; Kim et al. 1999; Bond and Lovely 2003; Marsili et al. 2008; Du et al. 2007) not only found evidence of electron transport between bacterial cells and their environment and helped to elucidate its mechanism, but also led to the development of important microbial fuel-cell applications (Figure 1).

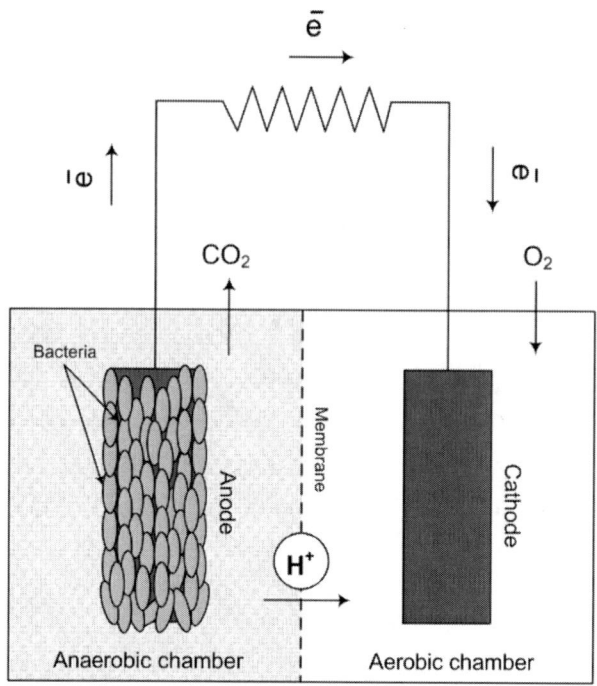

Figure 1. A typical two-chamber microbial fuel cell (Du, Li and Gu 2007).

It should be noted that the electrochemical activity of bacteria (e.g., *Shewanella putrefacient* or *Geobacter sulfurreducens*) is actually due to the enzymatic processes involving cytochrome (Kim et al. 1999), resulting in accumulation of electrons on the outer membrane. This excess of electrons serves as a donor for the electrophilic electron acceptors in the surrounding medium. While enzymatic processes also occur on the membranes of blood cells, in contrast to the bacterial processes these are intracellular and, therefore, do not lead to a spontaneous directed flow of electrons to the extracellular media. For blood cells, an appropriate potential gradient between the membrane and the environment is prerequisite to the activation of electron transport in a particular direction. Therefore, although interactions of an electrode with bacterial cells and with blood cells are largely analogous, significant differences also exist that must be considered, *viz.*, the respective unidirectional versus bidirectional nature of electron transport.

Most investigators point to the electrochemical nature of these interactions (e.g., Sawyer et al. 1964); however, it was not until recently (Tsivadze et al. 2017) that experimental evidence of the elementary act of electron transport between the electrode and blood cells was obtained. Therefore, experimental confirmation of electron transport between blood cells and foreign materials still presents a great deal of interest.

Earlier attempts to detect the electrochemical activity of blood cells experimentally and, thus, to corroborate the occurrence of electron transport in this system were unsuccessful. For example, Allen's investigation (1971) of the interaction between the mercury electrode and erythrocyte membranes suggested that electrooxidation of the sulfhydryl groups on the erythrocyte membrane occurred during the interaction of erythrocyte with the dropping mercury electrode (DME) according to Equation (1):

$$RSH + Hg \rightarrow RSHg + H^+ + e^- \tag{1}$$

Obviously, however, the reaction shown in Equation (1) could not proceed because deprotonation with the addition of mercury to the sulfhydryl group can only take place in the presence of oxygen or another oxidizing agent (Yamamoto et al. 2007), since the transfer of metallic mercury to the mercury ion is possible only in oxidizing media. However, Allen's experiments (1971) were carried out in the absence of oxidizing agents in solution.

Gingell and Fornes (1976; 1975) investigated the adhesion of erythrocytes to a polarized lead electrode in aqueous 1.2 mM sodium fluoride. Three characteristic ranges of electrode charge densities were identified: at positive charge densities ($+1.2 \times 10^3$ esu cm^{-2}), near zero charge, and in the slight negative range down to -5×10^3 esu cm^{-2}, the cells adhered to the electrode irreversibly. For negative charge densities between -5×10^3 esu cm^{-2} and -3×10^4 esu cm^{-2}, reversible adhesion occured; it could be overcome by increasing the negative charge density beyond -3×10^4 esu cm^{-2}, corresponding to the range of cell non-adhesion. However, no experimental evidence of electron transport was shown.

In the present work, the electrochemical behavior of erythrocytes in contact with certain electrically conductive materials was investigated in order to obtain experimental confirmation of electron transport in an electrochemical system comprising blood cells and foreign materials. Evidence of electrochemical activity of blood cells would strongly correlate with the existence of electron transport. To this end, polarization and coulometric measurements were made at platinum, carbonaceous, and optically transparent indium and tin oxide (ITO) electrodes. ITO electrodes were used to enable optical observation of erythrocyte morphology varying with electrode polarization.

EXPERIMENTAL

Polarization measurements were carried out in a three-electrode cell using a linear sweep of the potential at a rate of 10 mV/s from 0 mV to −1700 mV and from 0 mV to +1700 mV, with aqueous 0.15 M sodium chloride serving as the background electrolyte. The IPC Pro MF potentiostat (ZAO "Kronas," Russia) was used for electrochemical measurements. For measurements at the platinum and glassy carbon (GC) electrodes, magnetic stirring was utilized at 500 rpm; the selected rate provided sufficient intensity of stirring for the suspension, while at the same time minimizing injury to the blood cells (Simonyan et al. 1975).

Platinized titanium mesh was used as the auxiliary electrode for polarization measurements, with a saturated silver/silver chloride electrode as the reference electrode. Coulometric measurements at platinum and GC electrodes were carried out in a cell filled with a background electrolyte solution, with the electrode being polarized to a predetermined potential and held at this potential for 30 min. After 30 min, without interrupting the polarization, a suspension of erythrocytes or platelets was added to the background electrolyte solution to a content of 4.0×10^{12} cells/L and 2.2×10^{11} cells/L, respectively. Coulometric measurements were continued in the resulting suspension for 30 minutes.

Erythrocytes were obtained from the whole blood of apparently healthy donors and were triple-washed from plasma residue with physiological saline, with subsequent centrifugation on a CR 3.12 centrifuge (Jouan, France) at 1500g.

Hematological analysis of the cell content was carried out using the Ac·T diff 2 analyzer (Beckman Coulter, USA).

Deoxygenation of aqueous solutions was carried out via addition of sodium sulfite in order to avoid mechanical trauma of blood cells that would result from bubbling inert gas through the blood cell suspension. This method ensured the absence of dissolved oxygen that would interfere with oxidation/reduction observations: According to Durovic et al. (2015), the addition of sodium sulfite can completely remove oxygen from aqueous solutions on a time scale of 0.1 s to a few seconds. In order to remove 50% oxygen from erythrocytes, only 0.04 s is required (Simonyan 1975), with 11 min needed for full removal. However, full removal of oxygen from red blood cells requires the presence of carbon dioxide. These data are in agreement with other investigators' findings (Lawson et al. 1965; Mochizuki 1996).

To compute the amount of sodium sulfite needed to remove oxygen from the electrochemical cell, the amount of oxygen dissolved in the electrolyte was calculated. An assumption was made that all oxygen, including what is bound up in red blood cells, is released and must be removed by sodium sulfite.

The solubility of oxygen in water at 25°C of 8.3 mg/L, or 2.6×10^{-4} M (Battino et al. 1983), which corresponds to the total amount of oxygen in the background solution. Since the concentration of hemoglobin [MW = 66,800 g/mol] in blood is *ca.* 130 g/L (Turgeon 2005), or 1.94×10^{-3} M, with 4 mol oxygen per mole hemoglobin, the oxygen concentration in erythrocytes (and therefore total amount of oxygen in the suspended erythrocytes) is *ca.* 8.0×10^{-3} M.

However, in order to effect the full release of oxygen from the erythrocytes, the presence of carbon dioxide in the system is necessary. Indeed, according to the Verigo-Bohr effect (Nelson and Cox 2005), the equilibrium relationship between hemoglobin and erythrocyte oxygen in the human body depends on the pH of blood, as well as on the partial pressure of carbon dioxide (P_{CO_2}) in blood. *In vitro*, only part of the oxygen bound with hemoglobin can be released and dissolve in the solution surrounding the cell if there is no carbon dioxide present in the suspension.

Since the present work involved experiments performed *in vitro*, the suspension did not contain carbon dioxide, and the pH did not change during the experiment, the experimental conditions preclude the full removal of oxygen from the erythrocytes (Pokrovsky and Korot'ko 2003; Koolman and Roehm 2012). Therefore, the amount of oxygen that could be released upon the decomposition of the HbO_2 complex would be significantly less than the upper limit of the total oxygen amount in erythrocytes (which corresponds to full saturation of the hemoglobin). Thus, the assumptions made in the computation of the required sodium sulfite amount necessary for the full removal of oxygen corresponds to a significant excess of the sulfite ion in solution, thereby ensuring full removal of any dissolved oxygen.

The above considerations were corroborated by the analysis of the suspended erythrocytes in a background solution of 0.15 M NaCl in the presence and absence of 0.02 M Na_2SO_3 using a Stat Profile CCX blood gas analyzer (Nova Biomedical, USA). The contact time of the suspended erythrocytes with sodium sulfite was 30 minutes. The partial pressure of CO_2 in the erythrocyte suspension in the presence and absence of sodium sulfite was 7.2 mm Hg and 8.8 mm Hg, respectively. Compared to the normal range of CO_2 partial pressures of 40-50 mm Hg in erythrocyte suspensions, the present results correspond to a minimal partial pressure of CO_2 in the erythrocyte suspension. These data rule out the possibility of complete release of oxygen from the blood cells into the surrounding solution.

The presence of oxygen in the background electrolyte during the experiment was also measured by monitoring the excess amount of sodium sulfite in the solution via voltammetric data (utilizing its anodic oxidation peak). The likelihood of erythrocyte injury during contact with sodium sulfite was monitored by measuring the osmolarity of the solutions using an Osmomat 030 cryoscopic osmometer (Gonotec, Germany). With the addition of sodium sulfite to the background electrolyte to a concentration of 0.02 M, no significant changes in the osmolarity of the solution were observed. The initial 0.15 M NaCl solution exhibited an osmolarity of 308 mOsm/L, and an osmolarity of 314 mOsm/L was observed for the same solution containing 0.02 M Na_2SO_3.

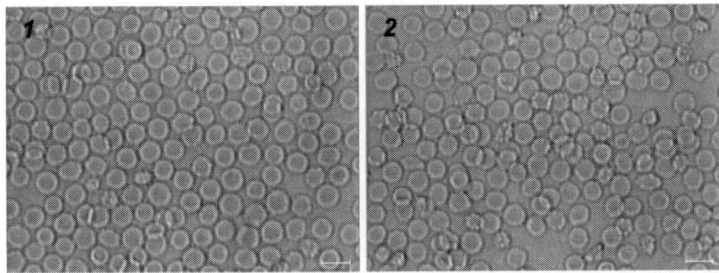

Figure 2. Microphotograph of the suspended erythrocytes in supporting electrolyte × 600: 1 – 0.15 M NaCl, 2 – 0.15 M NaCl + 0.02 M Na_2SO_3. Exposure time – 30 min.

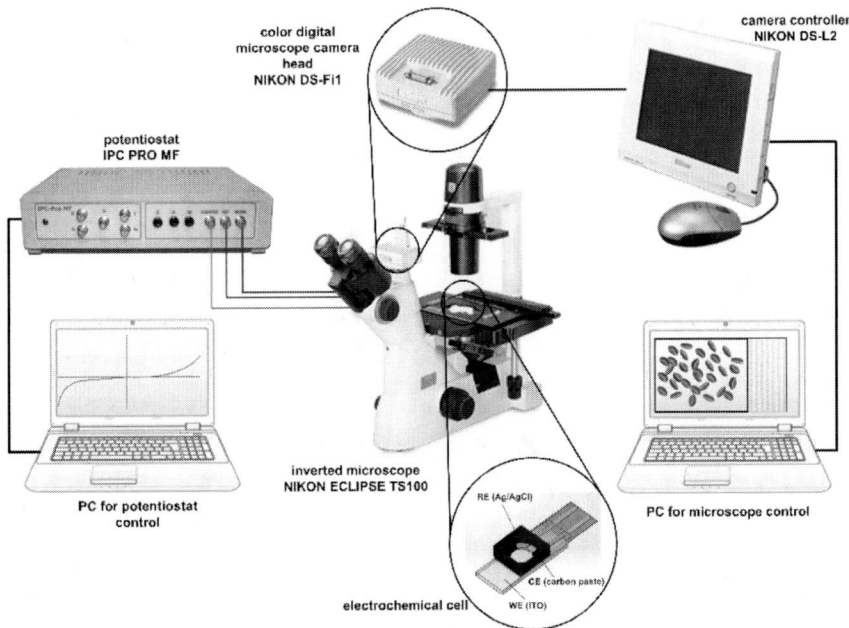

Figure 3. Three-electrode cell used for investigating erythrocyte morphology at optically transparent ITO electrodes.

Morphometric analysis of the erythrocytes following exposure to 0.15 M NaCl solutions with and without sodium sulfite for 30 min showed no change in the morphology of erythrocytes (Figure 2). This also corroborates the suitability of 0.02 M sodium sulfite solutions for full removal of dissolved oxygen from blood cell suspensions without causing cell damage. The traumatic effect of sodium sulfite on erythrocytes was not separately investigated. Polarization and coulometric measurements at cathodic potentials were carried out in the deoxygenated background electrolyte containing 0.15 M NaCl and 0.02 M Na_2SO_3, while it was not necessary to remove dissolved oxygen from the electrolyte for the polarization and coulometric measurements in the anodic range.

The effect of the potential of optically transparent ITO electrodes on erythrocyte morphology was investigated using in a three-electrode electrochemical cell (Figure 3) with a working ITO electrode (Sigma-Aldrich, USA) supported near the bottom of the electrochemical cell, a silver/silver chloride reference electrode, and a carbon paste auxiliary electrode. Morphological studies were performed utilizing an Eclipse TS100 inverted microscope (Nikon, Japan). Current-potential relationships were obtained via a linear potential sweep in range of potentials between −500 mV and +1400 mV.

Open-circuit potential (OCP) measurements were carried out on the platinum and activated carbon electrodes in 0.15 M NaCl solutions and erythrocytes suspensions in 0.15 M NaCl solutions.

RESULTS AND DISCUSSION

Addition of suspended erythrocytes to a deoxygenated solution of the background electrolyte (Figure 4, curve 1) resulted in the appearance of an electroreduction peak with a half-wave potential $E_{1/2} = -420$ mV (Figure 4, curve 2). The difference between this half-wave potential and the half-wave potential of the oxygen ionization process (which, according to our measurements under the same conditions, was $E_{1/2} = -340$ mV), was $\Delta E_{1/2} = -80$ mV.

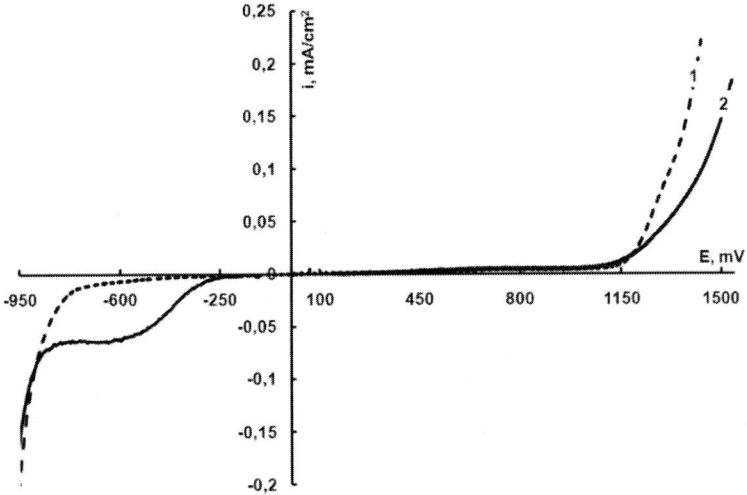

Figure 4. Polarization curves on the platinum electrode (scan rate 10 mV s^{-1}): 1 - background electrolyte, 2 – suspended erythrocytes in supporting electrolyte. Background electrolyte – 0.15 M NaCl (anodic potentials), 0.15 M NaCl + 0.02 M Na$_2$SO$_3$ (cathodic potentials).

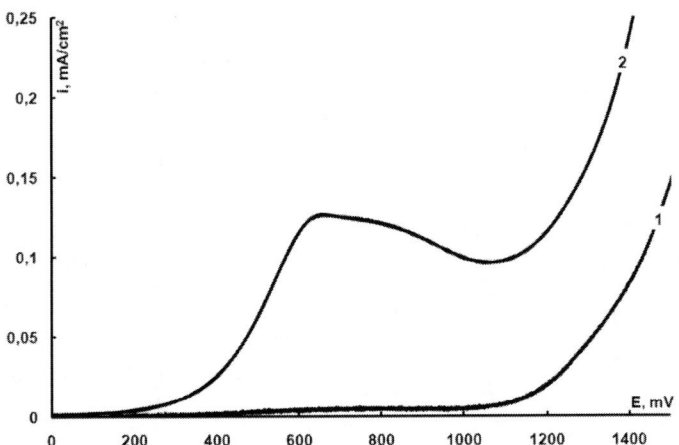

Figure 5. Anodic polarization curves at the platinum electrode (scan rate 10 mV s^{-1}): 1 – suspended erythrocytes in 0.15 M NaCl, 2 – suspended erythrocytes in 0.15 M NaCl + 0.02 M Na$_2$SO$_3$.

Anodic polarization measurements on the platinum electrode at a scan rate of 10 mV s^{-1} for both suspended erythrocytes in 0.15 M NaCl and suspended erythrocytes in 0.15 M NaCl with 0.02 M Na$_2$SO$_3$ added were performed to corroborate the absence of dissolved oxygen in the electrolyte containing sodium sulfite during the experiments. Polarization curves resulting from these measurements in the anodic potential region are shown in Figure 5. The oxidation peak of sodium sulfite on curve 2 indicates the consumption of dissolved oxygen upon the addition of the sodium sulfite and evidences the presence of dissolved oxygen after 30 min of polarization of the erythrocyte suspension using the background electrolyte alone (without sulfite addition).

The half-wave potential $E_{1/2} = -420$ mV observed upon addition of suspended erythrocytes to the background solution in the absence of dissolved oxygen (Figure 4, curve 2) shows the electrochemical activity of the blood cells.

Thus, direct experimental evidence of electron transport was obtained in the system comprising erythrocytes and the platinum electrode in the cathodic potential range. This electron transport could be rationalized as being due to the electroreduction of electron-acceptor groups present on the surface of the erythrocyte membrane.

An attempt was made to observe the electrooxidation process in the erythrocyte suspension, but this was not feasible via polarization measurements. The presence of the cathodic wave and the apparent absence of the anodic wave was rationalized by considering the ratio of electron-acceptor (electrophilic) and electron-donor (nucleophilic) functional groups on the surface of the erythrocyte membrane. Indeed, if the quantity of the electrophilic groups is several orders of magnitude greater than the quantity of the nucleophilic functionalities on the membrane surface, the current required for electrooxidation processes would likewise be orders of magnitude smaller than that for electroreduction. Therefore, if the polarization measurements lacked sufficient sensitivity, the electrochemical behavior of suspended erythrocytes on the platinum electrode could be investigated via coulometric measurements. These measurements proved to be very effective. The occurrence of both electroreduction and electrooxidation processes in a deoxygenated background electrolyte containing suspended erythrocytes was experimentally confirmed.

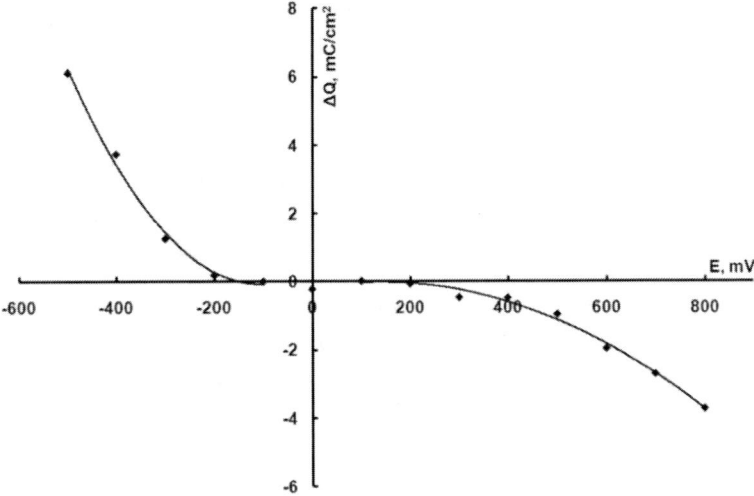

Figure 6. Coulometric measurements for suspended erythrocytes (4×10^{12} cells/L) at the platinum electrode in 0.15 M NaCl (anodic potentials) and 0.15 M NaCl + 0.02 M Na_2SO_3 (cathodic potentials).

The results of coulometric measurements shown in Figure 6 show that the measured values of the charge depend on the polarization potential of the platinum electrode. These data revealed an increase in the intensity of, respectively, electroreduction when the potential shifted in the negative direction, and electrooxidation, when the electrode potential shifted in the positive direction. This corroborated the occurrence of electron transport between the erythrocyte cells and the platinum electrode, owing to the electroreduction and electrooxidation reactions determining the respective directionality of such transport (i.e., from the electrode to blood cell membranes or vice versa). In terms of surface chemistry of the membrane, electrons transport from the electrode to the membrane corresponds to the electroreduction of electron-acceptor groups on the membrane surface, and, contrariwise for electron transport in the opposite direction (from electron-donor groups to the electrode) indicates the electrooxidation of membrane surface functionalities. It should be noted that the presence of such functional groups on the surface of blood cell membranes has been shown in a number of investigations (Seaman 1973; Gwynne and Tanford 1970; Reglinsky et al. 1988). In contrast to the above charge transport phenomena for blood cells, only the unidirectional electron transport – from the microbial cell through the membrane to the electrode – can occur for microbial cells (Du et al. 2007).

As shown in Figure 6, in the potential range from −150 mV to +200 mV the electrode charge remains essentially unchanged, indicating the absence of electrochemical processes in this potential range. Thus, a range of potentials where the working electrode is indifferent toward the erythrocytes can be identified via coulometric measurements in the erythrocyte suspension, providing an experimental electrochemical first approximation of the potential range of hemocompatibility for foreign materials.

In order to determine the influence of the electrode material on the electrochemical behavior of erythrocytes, GC was selected as a chemically inert electrode material (Van der Linden and Dieker 1980). Figure 7 shows the polarization curves on the GC electrode at a scan rate of 10 mV·s^{-1} in the background electrolyte (curve 1) and also for suspended erythrocytes in the background electrolyte (curve 2). The half-wave potential after the addition of erythrocytes to the deoxygenated background electrolyte is observed at $E_{1/2}$ = −770 mV (curve 2), while the half-wave potential corresponding to the process of dissolved oxygen electroreduction was observed at $E_{1/2}$ = −630 mV under the same conditions. The difference between these values is +140 mV, indicating that the peak with the half-wave potential value of $E_{1/2}$ = −770 mV correlated with the reduction of electron-acceptor groups on the surface of the erythrocyte membrane that is similar to the electroreduction of electron-acceptor groups on platinum. The observed effect can serve as experimental corroboration of the occurrence of electron transport between suspended erythrocytes and the GC electrode.

The results of coulometric measurements for the system comprising suspended erythrocytes and the GC electrode in the cathodic and anodic potential ranges are shown in Figures 8 and 9, respectively.

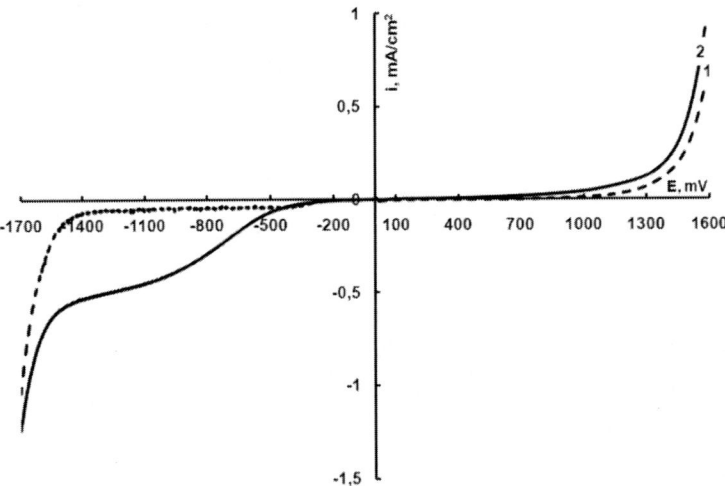

Figure 7. Polarization curves on the GC electrode (scan rate 10 mV s^{-1}): 1 - supporting electrolyte, 2 – erythrocyte suspension in background electrolyte. Background electrolyte – 0.15 M NaCl (anodic potentials), 0.15 M NaCl + 0.02 M Na_2SO_3 (cathodic potentials).

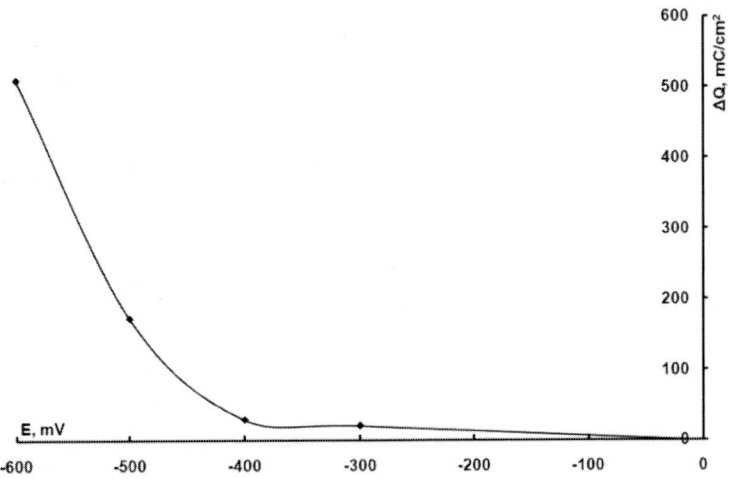

Figure 8. Coulometric measurements for suspended erythrocytes (4×10^{12} cells/L) in 0.15 M NaCl + 0.02 M Na_2SO_3 at the GC electrode at cathodic potentials.

The figures show that the difference between the charge expended for the electroreduction of the erythrocyte suspension in the background electrolyte and the charge that passed through the background electrolyte without blood cells begins to increase at the GC potential $E = -100$ mV (Figure 8). These data experimentally corroborate the occurrence of electron transport from the electrode to the erythrocyte and, thus, of the electroreduction reaction of functional groups on the erythrocyte membranes in the presence of suspended erythrocytes.

Thus, electron transport between suspended erythrocytes and the electrode surface, accompanied by electrooxidation or electroreduction, was shown to occur on the platinum and GC electrodes. Moreover, the data shown in Figures 8 and 9 demonstrate that there are potential ranges where the erythrocytes do not interact with the surface of the electrode (i.e., the "indifference range"). For the GC electrode, this "indifference range" towards erythrocytes is in the potential range between -100 mV and $+150$ mV. As detailed above, this range corresponding to the indifference of the electrode towards erythrocytes can be utilized to determine the hemocompatibility of any electrically conductive material by comparing it to the open-circuit potential of the material in the same environment.

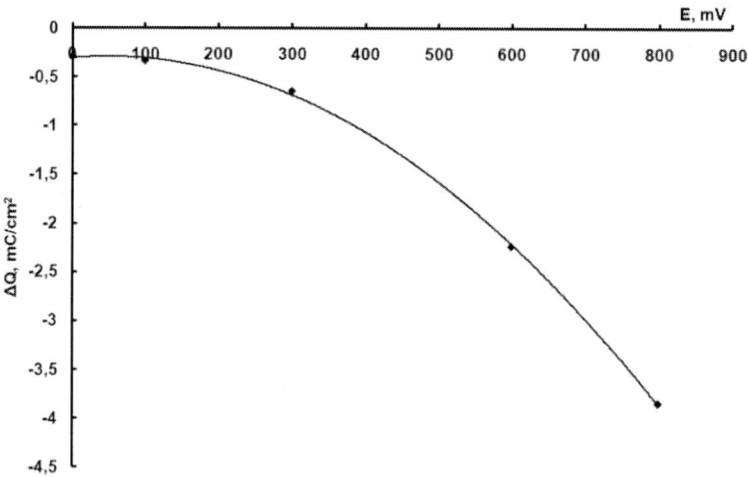

Figure 9. Coulometric measurements for suspended erythrocytes (4×10^{12} cells/L) in 0.15 M NaCl at the GC electrode at anodic potentials.

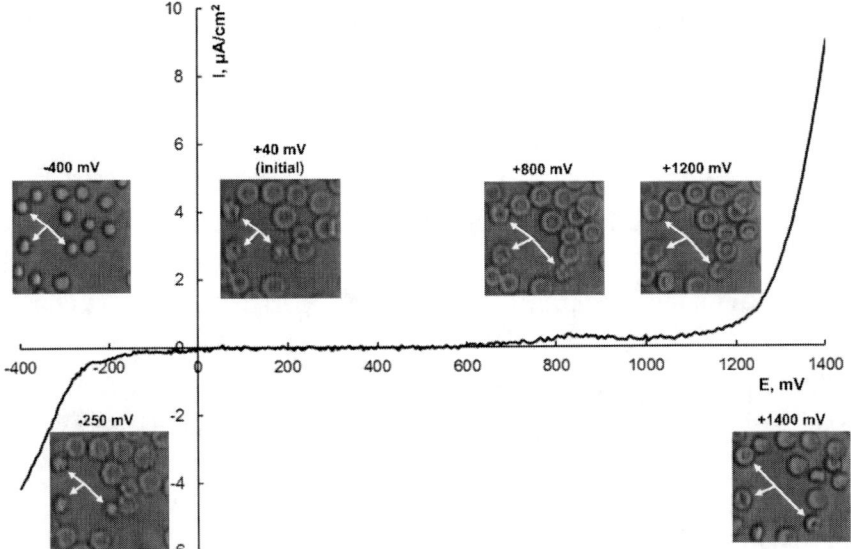

Figure 10. Erythrocyte morphology for various ITO electrode potentials in 0.15 M NaCl.

It is worth noting that the absolute value of the charge transferred in the course of electroreduction of suspended erythrocytes on the GC electrode after 30 minutes is greater than the absolute value of the charge transferred in the electroreduction of suspended erythrocytes at the platinum electrode during the same amount of time. This important effect highlights the influence of the nature of the electrode material on the kinetics of the electrode process. The potential range on the GC electrode corresponding to electrode indifference (i.e., no interaction of blood cells with the electrode) is similar to those previously observed for activated carbons (Goldin et al. 2006).

The use of optically transparent ITO electrodes enabled the use of light microscopy to detect morphological changes in erythrocytes in real time depending on the applied electrode potential.

The erythrocyte morphometry data were obtained at the ITO electrode in a potential range between –400 and +1400 mV (Figure 10). The initial normal morphology of the red blood cells (discocytes) degenerates into various pathological morphologies with changes in electrode potential.

Importantly, each of the morphologies occurred in a specific potential range. For instance, all discocytes transform into echinocytes at potentials more negative than –350 mV. With increasingly negative potentials below this value, the entire sample of red blood cells gradually takes on a spherocyte morphology.

For anodic potentials up to +600 mV, no changes in cell morphologies were detected. However, a very important effect was observed at potentials between +600 and +1200 mV, where the degenerative erythrocyte forms (echinocyte) changed back to the normal discocytes (Figure 11 – marked by the arrow). Finally, for potentials more positive than +1300 mV, normal discocytes transferred into a different pathological form (stomatocytes).

It is important that the normal-to- degenerative form transitions were reversible: when the external electrode polarization was switched off, the cells returned to their initial, normal morphological form.

Additionally, the observed electrochemical activity of the erythrocytes at platinum and CG electrodes in the anodic potential range was observed at the ITO electrode as well (Figure 11). The limiting electrooxidation currents were found to follow a linear dependence on the suspended erythrocyte concentration in the range between 8×10^9 and 8×10^{11} cells/L.

According to the data published on the structure and composition of blood cell membranes (Seaman 1973; Gwynne and Tanford 1970; Reglinsky et al. 1988), the electron donors correspond to sulfhydryl or similar functionalities of amino acids, while the electron-acceptor functional groups of amino acids are disulfides, such as those found in glycoproteins that make up the cell membrane.

Hypothetically, the transport of electrons between erythrocytes and the electrode may also occur without external polarization due to the difference in the charge densities on the cell membrane and the electrode surface. This hypothesis was corroborated via measurements of OCP of the platinum electrode and FAS brand activated carbon immersed in 0.15 M aqueous sodium chloride, both prior to and following the addition of suspended erythrocytes to the electrolyte (Figure 12-a and b).

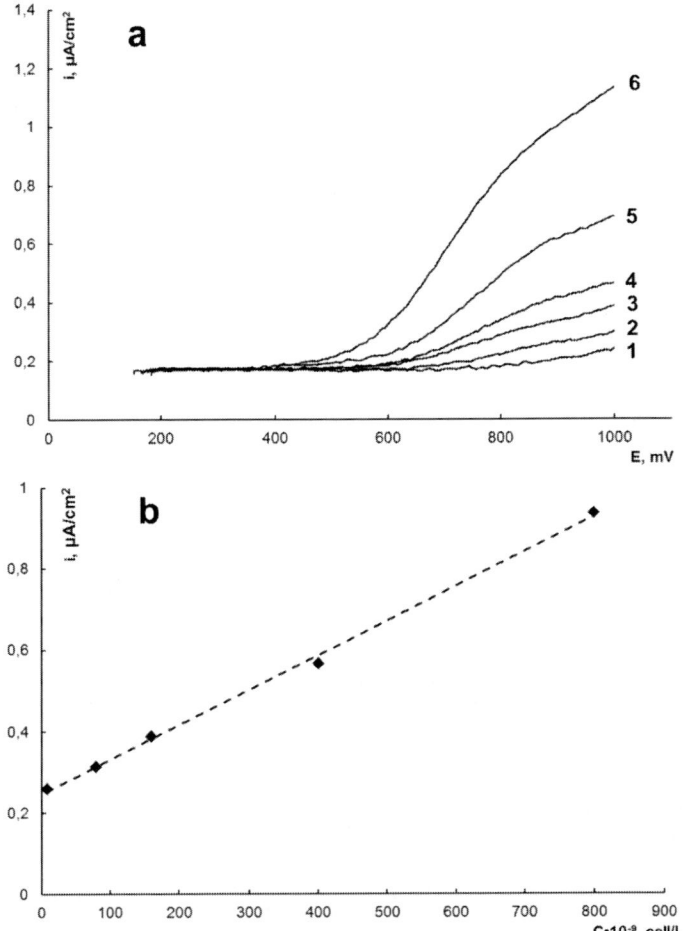

Figure 11. Polarization curves in the erythrocyte suspension (a) (cells/L): 1 – background (0.15 M NaCl), 2 – 8×10^9, 3 – 8×10^{10}, 4 – 1.6×10^{11}, 5 – 4×10^{11}, 6 – 8×10^{11}; current densities measured at $E = +850$ mV vs. cell concentration (b).

As shown in Figure 12-a, the addition of suspended erythrocytes to the background electrolyte (aqueous 0.15 M NaCl) leads to significant shifts in the OCP of the platinum electrode in the negative direction ($\Delta E = -106$ mV). This OCP shift reflects a change in the magnitude of the surface charge density of the platinum electrode. Such phenomena can be caused only by the electron transport from the surface of the cell membrane to the electrode.

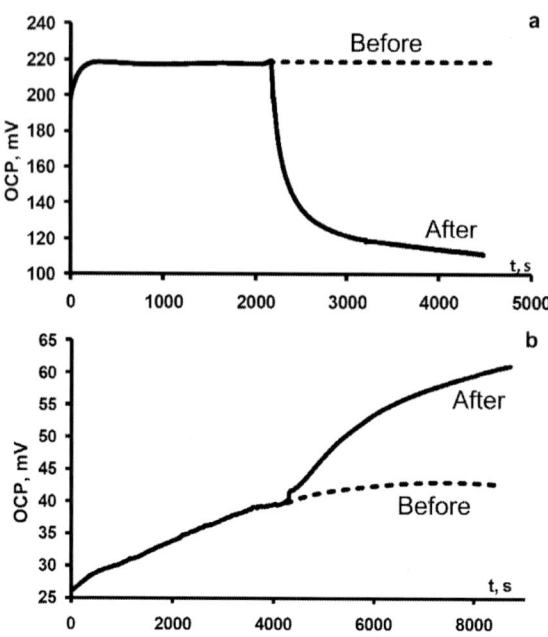

Figure 12. Open-circuit potentials of electrodes immersed in 0.15 M NaCl before and after the addition of suspended erythrocytes: (a) using the Pt electrode and (b) using a FAS activated carbon brand electrode.

The same phenomenon, but with the opposite sign, is observed when activated carbon (FAS brand) is used as the electrode (see Figure 12-b). The addition of suspended erythrocyte into the background electrolyte leads to an OCP shift of the activated carbon in the positive direction ($\Delta E = +21$ mV), indicating that the electron transport occurs from the activated carbon surface to the cell membrane.

Differences in the absolute value of the potential shift on the activated carbon electrode in comparison with that on the platinum electrode can be rationalized by noting the significant difference between the surfaces areas of the two electrodes, measuring 300 m^2 and 1.6×10^{-6} m^2 for activated carbon and platinum, respectively. Indeed, the smooth platinum surface is entirely visible, while the specific surface area of the activated carbon brand FAS is about 1000 $m^2 \cdot g^{-1}$. At the same time, the charge density of the erythrocyte membrane surface is constant, and the number of blood cells used in both experiments was on the same order of magnitude.

Thus, experimental evidence was found for the occurrence of electron transport between the electrode and erythrocytes. A correlation between the electrode potential and the morphologies of red blood cells was established, with both reversible and irreversible potential-dependent morphologic changes occurring. The observed effects are useful for the development of diagnostic methods of erythrocyte quality control and, possibly, methods for improving their quality after prolonged storage via electrode polarization to certain potential ranges.

CONCLUSION

Polarization measurements showed that human erythrocytes are electrochemically active, i.e., they undergo electroreduction and electrooxidation at platinum, glassy carbon, and optically transparent ITO electrodes. Coulometric measurements also corroborated the occurrence of electron transport between the erythrocytes and the electrodes. Electron transport was shown to occur from the surface of the electrode to the cell membrane, as well as in the opposite direction. It was hypothesized that the electrochemical transformations occur in nucleophilic (electron-donor) and electrophilic (electron-acceptor) functional groups of the amino acids that make on the surface of cell membranes. OCP measurements showed that the transport of electrons was dependent upon the ratio of the charge densities of cell membrane surface and the foreign-material surface, both in the presence and absence of external polarization. Coulometric measurements were utilized to establish the potential ranges corresponding to the indifference of the electrode with respect to the blood cells, allowing the use of coulometry to evaluate the hemocompatibility of electrically conductive materials. Both reversible and irreversible transformations of erythrocyte morphology caused by changes of the potential of the foreign material were observed and investigated.

REFERENCES

[1] Abramson, H. A. 1934. *Electrokinetic Phenomena and Their Application to Biology and Medicine*. New York: The Chemical Catalog Company Inc.

[2] Abramson, H. A., Furchgott, R. F. and Ponder, E. 1939. "The Electrophoretic Mobility of Rabbit Erythrocytes and Ghosts." *Journal of General Physiology* 22(4): 545-553.

[3] Allen, M. J. 1971. "Electrochemical Behavior of Blood. I. A Voltammetric Study of Metabolizing Erythrocytes." *Collection of Czechoslovak Chemical Communications* 36: 658-663.

[4] Battino, R., Rettich, T. R. and Tominaga, T. 1983. "The Solubility of Oxygen and Ozone in Liquids." *Journal of Physical and Chemical Reference Data* 12(2): 163-178.

[5] Bond, D. R. and Lovley, D. R. 2003. "Electricity Production by Geobacter sulfurreducens Attached to Electrodes." *Applied and Environmental Microbiology* 69(3): 1548-1555.

[6] Chepurov, A. K. and Mertsalova N. N. 1978. "The Interrelationships Between Blood Coagulation, the Charge and the Surface Roughness" I. M. *Sechenov Journal of Physiology of the USSR* 64 (11): 1559-1566.

[7] Delaney, G. M., Bennetto, H. P., Mason, J. R., Roller, S. D., Stirling, J. L. and Thurston, C. F. 1984. "Electron-transfer Coupling in Microbial Fuel Cells. 2. Performance of Fuel Cells Containing Selected Microorganism – Mediator - Substrate Combinations." *Journal of Chemical Technology and Biotechnology* 34(1): 13-27.

[8] Du, Z., Li, H. and Gu, T. 2007. "A State of the Art Review on Microbial Fuel Cells: A Promising Technology for Wastewater Treatment and Bioenergy." *Biotechnology Advances* 25: 464-482 (2007).

[9] Durovic, A. D., Stojanovic, Z. S., Kravic, S. Z., Suturovic, Z. J., Brezo, T. Z., Grahovac, N. L. and Milanovic, C. D. 2015. "A Comparison of Different Methods to Remove Dissolved Oxygen:

Application to the Electrochemical Determination of Imidacloprid." *Acta Periodica Technologica* 46: 149-155.

[10] Evseev, A. K., Mikhailov, I. P., Popova, T. S., Smirnov, K. N., Kruglikov, S. S. and Goldin, M. M. 2014. "The Use of Rhodium Coating as an Insoluble Anode for the Endovascular Embolization." *Eletroplating and Surface Treatment* 22 (1): 45-50 (2014) [in Russian].

[11] Furchgott, R. F. and Ponder, E. 1941. "Electrophoretic studies on Human Red Blood Cells." *Journal of General Physiology* 24(4): 447-457.

[12] Gingell, D. and Fornes, J. A. 1975. "Demonstration of Intermolecular Forces in Cell Adhesion Using a New Electrochemical Technique." *Nature* 256: 210-211.

[13] Gingell, D. and Fornes, J. A. 1976. "Interaction of Red Blood Cells with a Polarized Electrode: Evidence of Long-range Intermolecular Forces." *Biophysical Journal* 16(10): 1131-1153.

[14] Goldin, M. M., Luzhnikov, E. A. and Suslova, I. M. 1980. "The Influence of Electrochemical Characteristics of the Sorbent on Blood Cells Concentration During Hemosorption." *Russian Journal of Electrochemistry* 16(11): 1667-1669 [in Russian].

[15] Goldin, M. M., Volkov, A. G., Goldfarb, Y. S. and Goldin, Michael M. 2006. "Electrochemical Aspects of Hemosorption." *Journal of Electrochemical Society* 153(8): J91-J99.

[16] Gwynne, J. T. and Tanford, C. A. 1970. "A Polypeptide Chain of Very High Molecular Weight from Red Blood Cell Membranes." *Journal of Biological Chemistry* 245(12): 3269-3273.

[17] Ji, C., Guglielmi, G. and Chen, H. 1997. "Endovascular Electrocoagulation: Concept, Technique, and Experimental Results." *American Journal of Neuroradiology* 18(9):1669-78.

[18] Kharamonenko, S. S. and Rakityanskaya, A. A. 1974 *Electrophorez Kletok Krovi v Norme i Patologii* [*Electrophoresis of Blood Cells in Norm and Pathology*]. Minsk: Belarus Publications [in Russian].

[19] Kim, B. H., Kim, H. J., Hyun, M. S. and Park, D. H. 1999. "Direct Electrode Reaction of Fe(III)-reducing Bacterium, Shewanella

putrefaciens." *Journal of Microbiology and Biotechnology* 9(2): 127-131.

[20] Koolman, J. and Roehm, K. H. 2012. *Color Atlas of Biochemistry*, 3^d ed. New York: Thieme.

[21] Lawson, W. H., Holland, R. A. B. and Forster, R. E. 1965. "Effect of Temperature on Deoxygenation Rate of Human Red Cells." *Journal of Applied Physiology* 20(5): 912-918.

[22] Luzhnikov, E. A., Goldin, M. M. and Suslova, I. M. 1980. "The Potential of the Sorbent and Blood Cells Safety." *Farmatsiya* 3: 65-66 [in Russian].

[23] Marsili, E., Baron, D. B., Shikhare, I. D., Coursolle, D., Gralnick, J.A. and Bond, D. R. 2008. "Shewanella Secretes Flavins That Mediate Extracellular Electron Transfer." *Proceedings of the National Academy of Sciences of the United States of America* 105(10): 3968-3973.

[24] Martin, J. G., Afshar A., Kapllit, M. G., Chopra, P. S., Srinivasan, S. and Sawyer, P. N. 1968. "Implantation Studies With Some Nonmetallic Prostheses." *Transactions - American Society for Artificial Internal Organs* 14: 78-81.

[25] Michelson, A. D. 2012. Platelets, 3rd ed., London: Academic Press.

[26] Mochizuki, M. 1966. "On the Velocity of Oxygen Dissociation of Human Hemoglobin and Red Cell." *The Japanese Journal of Physiology* 16: 649-657.

[27] Nelson, D. L. and Cox, M. M. 2005. *Lehninger Principles of Biochemistry*, 4th ed. W. H. Freeman & Co.

[28] Pokrovsky, V. M. and Korot'ko, G.F. 2003. *Phiziologiya cheloveka* [*Human physiology*]. Moscow: Meditsina.

[29] Reglinsky, J., Hoey, S., Smith, W. E., Sturrock, R. D. 1988. "Cellular Response to Oxidative Stress at Sulfhydryl Group Receptor Sites on the Erythrocyte Membrane." *Journal of Biological Chemistry* 263:12360-12366.

[30] Sawyer, P. N. 1983. "The Relationship between Surface Charge (Potential Characteristics) of the Vascular Interface and Thrombosis." *Annals of the New York Academy of Sciences* 416(1): 561-583.

[31] Sawyer, P. N. 1984. "Electrode-Biologic Tissue Interactions at Interfaces - A Review" *Biomaterials, Medical Devices and Artificial Organs* 12: 161-196.

[32] Sawyer, P. N. and Pate, J. W. 1953. "Bio-electric Phenomena as an Etiologic Factor in Intravascular Thrombosis." *The American journal of physiology* 175(1): 103-107.

[33] Sawyer, P. N., Brattain, W. H., and Boddy, P. J. 1964. "Electrochemical Precipitation of Human Blood Cells and its Possible Relation to Intravascular Thrombosis." *Proceedings of the National Academy of Sciences of the United States of America* 51: 428-432.

[34] Sawyer, P. N., Ogoniak, J. C. and Boddy, P. J. 1967. "The Interaction Between Human Erythrocytes and Metal Surfaces." *Surgery* 61(3): 448-454.

[35] Sawyer, P. N., Srinivasan S., Stanczewski, B., Ramasamy, N. and Ramsey, W. 1974. "Electrochemical Aspects of Thrombogenesis - Bioelectrochemistry Old and New." *Journal of Electrochemical Society* 121(7): 221C-234C.

[36] Sawyer, P. N., Wu, K. T., Wesolowski, S. A., Brattain, W. H. and Boddy, P. J. 1965. "Electrochemical Precipitation of Blood Cells on Metal Electrodes: an Aid in the Selection of Vascular Prostheses?" *Proceedings of the National Academy of Sciences of the United States of America* 53: 294-300.

[37] Seaman, G. V. F. 1973. "The Surface Chemistry of the Erythrocyte and Thrombocyte Membrane." *Journal of Cellular Biochemistry* 1(4-5): 437-447.

[38] Seaman, G. V. F. and Vassar, P. S. 1966. "Changes in the Electrokinetic Properties of Platelets during their Aggregation." *Archives of Biochemistry and Biophysics* 117(1):10-17.

[39] Simonyan, K. S., Gutiontova, K. P., Tsurinova, E. G., 1975. *Posmertnaya Krov' v Aspekte Transfuziologii*. [*Death Blood' in the Aspect of Transfusiology*]. Moscow: Meditsina [in Russian].

[40] Srinivasan, S. and Sawyer, P. N. 1970. "Role of Surface Charge of the Blood Vessel Wall, Blood Cells, and Prosthetic Materials in

Intravascular Thrombosis." *Journal of Colloid and Interface Science* 32(3): 456-463.

[41] Tsivadze, A. Y., Khubutiya, M. S., Goroncharovskaya, I. V., Evseev, A. K., Goldin, Michael M., Borovkova, N. V., Batishchev, O. V. and Goldin, Mark M. 2017. "Electron Transport and Morphological Changes in the Electrode/Erythrocyte System." *Mendeleev Communications* 27(2): 183-185.

[42] Turgeon, M. L. 2005. *Clinical Hematology: theory and procedures*, 4th ed. Philadelphia: Lippincott Williams & Wilkins.

[43] Van der Linden, W. E. and Dieker, J. W. 1980. "Glassy Carbon as Electrode Material in Electro - analytical Chemistry." *Analytica Chimica Acta* 119(1): 1-24.

[44] Yamamoto, M., Charoenrak, T., Pan-Hou, H., Nakano, A., Apilux, A. and Tabata, M. 2007. "Electrochemical Behaviors of Sulfhydryl Compounds in the Presence of Elemental Mercury." *Chemosphere* 69(4): 534-539.

INDEX

A

actin, 24, 27, 35, 45, 66, 67, 79
AFM, 102, 103
animal blood, 107
animal erythrocytes, 69, 88, 89, 91, 119
ankyrin, 24, 26, 27, 34, 66, 67
annexin V binding test, 96
anti-inflammatory drug, 73, 89, 97
autologous, 59, 60, 63, 76, 87, 89, 107, 110, 111, 121, 126
average diameter, 63, 95

B

band 3, 24, 26, 27, 28, 29, 34, 35, 45, 46, 65, 66, 67, 77, 79, 80, 81, 108, 114, 115, 124
biochemical properties, 95
biological activity, 83, 114
biologically active compound, 75
biomimetic delivery platform, 63, 117
bovine erythrocytes, 85, 90, 91, 93, 96, 125, 127, 128

C

cellular carriers, 68
cellular hitchhiking strategy, 62
cholesterol, 65, 73, 96, 127, 128
colloidal properties, 85, 120
coulometry, 155
cytoskeleton, 8, 24, 26, 34, 65, 96, 121, 124, 127, 132

D

dexamethasone-sodium phosphate, 89
diffraction, 95, 102
diffusion, 25, 68, 81, 95, 97, 101, 103
diffusion and partition coefficient, 95, 97
dosage, 107
dosage frequency, 107
drug carriers, x, 58, 62, 63, 64, 68, 84, 89, 99, 107, 109, 113
drug content, 68, 71, 98
drug delivery, v, vii, x, 57, 58, 61, 62, 64, 68, 69, 84, 87, 88, 90, 95, 98, 106, 108, 109, 113, 115, 116, 118, 119, 120, 121, 122, 123, 124, 126, 128, 130
drug delivery systems, v, vii, x, 57, 58, 61, 62, 64, 68, 88, 90, 95, 98

drug pharmacokinetics, 63
drug release, vii, x, 58, 68, 104
drug release profile, vii, x, 58, 68, 104
drug vehicles, 64, 94, 119

E

echinocyte, 95, 152
electrochemical potential, 137
encapsulation, x, 58, 60, 61, 64, 67, 69, 70, 71, 72, 73, 74, 75, 76, 77, 86, 90, 92, 95, 97, 98, 99, 101, 102, 103, 106, 109, 110, 112, 116, 120, 121, 127, 130, 131
encapsulation efficacy, 70
encapsulation efficiency, 75, 100, 101
encapsulation methods, 71, 74, 76
encapsulation potential, 70
encapsulation process, 70, 77, 98, 99
enzymes, ix, 22, 35, 36, 37, 39, 40, 49, 61, 66, 75, 83, 100, 112
enzymopathies, ix, 22, 23, 25, 35, 36, 40
erythrocyte disorders, v, ix, 21, 22, 25, 33, 41, 42, 44
erythrocyte ghosts, 58, 60, 63, 83, 85, 86, 87, 88, 89, 91, 92, 93, 94, 95, 96, 97, 99, 101, 102, 103, 105, 106, 107, 110, 112, 115, 116, 118, 126, 131
erythrocyte membrane, v, vii, x, 24, 25, 26, 28, 30, 34, 46, 48, 57, 58, 60, 61, 63, 64, 65, 67, 68, 69, 70, 71, 72, 76, 80, 83, 85, 86, 87, 88, 89, 95, 96, 97, 100, 101, 105, 106, 108, 109, 113, 114, 115, 117, 119, 120, 124, 129, 139, 146, 148, 150, 154, 158
erythrocyte membrane templated microcapsules, 88
erythrocyte shape, ix, 22, 26, 34, 80, 95, 124
erythrocyte swelling, 74, 77, 78, 79, 80, 98, 125, 128
erythropoiesis, vii, viii, 1, 2, 3, 4, 7, 8, 9, 10, 11, 13, 17, 18, 19, 21, 23, 49

extracellular hemoglobin, 93

F

FE-SEM, 95, 102
flow cytometry, 9, 92, 124
foreign materials, x, 133, 135, 139, 140, 148

G

gradual hypotonic hemolysis, 93, 94, 96, 97, 98, 102, 119

H

hemoglobin, viii, ix, 5, 8, 21, 22, 23, 24, 25, 27, 29, 30, 31, 32, 33, 41, 42, 43, 47, 48, 60, 64, 67, 68, 69, 72, 77, 81, 83, 87, 90, 93, 94, 97, 102, 104, 108, 110, 119, 123, 125, 127, 130, 131, 141, 142, 158
hemoglobin content, ix, 22, 41, 42, 68, 98, 104
hemoglobinopathies, ix, 22, 23, 25, 30, 47, 49
hemolytic hole, 77, 80, 81, 82, 83, 98
heterologous erythrocytes, 89
hPSCs, viii, 1, 2, 3, 4, 5, 6, 7, 8, 9, 10, 11, 12, 13
HSC-independent, 2, 3, 7, 8, 11, 12, 13
human erythrocytes, 3, 6, 48, 59, 62, 64, 65, 68, 69, 75, 77, 87, 89, 92, 105, 108, 113, 115, 116, 126, 127, 155, 159
hypotonic buffer, 60, 72, 74, 75, 93
hypotonic conditions, 76, 77, 81, 92, 124
hypotonic dialysis, 75, 76, 98, 114, 122
hypotonic dilution, 73, 74, 75, 98
hypotonic hemolysis, 72, 73, 92, 94, 96, 97, 98
hypotonic pre-swelling, 74, 87, 98

Index

I

immune system, 63, 86, 107
in vitro characterization, 68
inflammatory/malignant diseases, 59
interaction, v, x, 18, 45, 96, 105, 133, 135, 139, 151, 157, 159
inter-individual variations, 98
isotonic phosphate buffers, 101

L

laser diffraction method, 95, 102
layer-by-layer assembly, 88, 122
life span, viii, 21, 64, 68, 75, 86
lipid bilayer, 24, 26, 66, 72, 78, 80, 81, 118, 124
lipid membrane composition, 68, 91
liposomes, 59, 64, 71, 85, 100, 114, 117, 118, 128

M

macrophage uptake, 63
major protein fractions, 95
mammalian erythrocyte membrane, 63
mass spectrometry, 99
mechanisms of pore formation, 83, 107
membrane disorders, 23, 25, 26, 45, 46
membrane integrity, 35, 60
membrane surface, 66, 85, 86, 146, 147, 155
microhematocrit method, 92
microscopy methods, 68
modeling considerations, 76, 124
mononuclear phagocyte system, 67, 84
morphology, v, xi, 31, 42, 64, 68, 81, 95, 102, 103, 133, 134, 140, 143, 144, 151, 155

N

nanoerythrosomes, x, 58, 61, 63, 84, 86, 106, 108, 112, 113, 120, 123
nanoparticles, x, 58, 61, 62, 63, 86, 106, 109, 111, 113, 116, 117, 121, 128

O

opening of pores on erythrocyte membrane, 69
optimal procedure condition, 69
osmolarity, 90, 142
osmosis, 69, 71, 72, 76, 83, 114
osmosis based methods, 69, 71, 72
osmosis-based drug encapsulation, 76, 83, 114
osmotic fragility, 28, 29, 33, 39, 43, 68, 91, 93, 107
osmotic fragility analysis, 68, 93
osmotic hemolysis, 67, 112
osmotic resistance, viii, 22, 28, 90, 91
osmotic shock, 95

P

partition, 95, 97
pharmacodynamics, 63, 116
phase contrast microscopy, 68, 94
phosphatidylserine, 34, 65, 71, 96
phospholipid bilayer, 67, 96
phospholipids, 48, 65, 96, 100
polarization measurements, 140, 145, 146
porcine erythrocytes, 90, 91, 93, 94, 95, 96, 99
preclinical studies, 89
prolonged release, 60, 63, 89, 105, 107, 113, 131

R

red blood cells, vii, viii, x, 14, 15, 16, 17, 19, 21, 23, 41, 45, 46, 48, 58, 64, 67, 69, 91, 94, 109, 110, 114, 116, 117, 120, 122, 123, 125, 126, 127, 128, 134, 141, 151, 155, 157
relaxation time, 77
release kinetics, 99, 103
resealed erythrocyte, 60, 69, 115, 117
resealing the pores of the resultant cellular carriers, 69
residual hemoglobin, 103, 104
roughness, 95, 102, 156

S

SDS-PAGE, 95
shape, vii, viii, 21, 22, 25, 27, 31, 32, 41, 42, 45, 64, 66, 68, 72, 85, 91, 95, 102, 118
size, ix, 22, 23, 41, 42, 68, 85, 86, 87, 88, 91, 95, 96, 97, 102, 104
size distribution, 68, 92, 95
slaughterhouse blood, 89, 90, 92, 93, 94, 97, 113, 119, 129, 131
sodium, 89
spectrin, 24, 26, 27, 34, 35, 46, 65, 66, 67, 79, 80
structural integrity, 77, 80
surface morphology e, 68
surface potential, 68
swelling degree, 90

T

targeted delivery, x, 58, 59, 87, 89, 96, 107, 115, 118
the inside-out, 96
theoretical models, 76
tonicity, 73, 74, 75, 77, 79, 81, 94
toxicity, 107
toxicity reduction, 107

V

volume, ix, 22, 25, 28, 29, 33, 41, 47, 64, 68, 72, 73, 75, 78, 79, 80, 82, 84, 90, 91, 93, 95, 97, 118

X

xenogeneic, 88, 89

Related Nova Publications

BENIGN AND MALIGNANT DISORDERS OF LARGE GRANULAR LYMPHOCYTES: DIAGNOSTIC AND THERAPEUTIC PEARLS

EDITORS: Ling Zhang, M.D. and Lubomir Sokol, M.D., Ph.D.

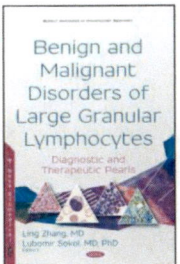

SERIES: Recent Advances in Hematology Research

BOOK DESCRIPTION: Natural killer (NK) cells are important effector cells of innate immune system implicated in many physiological processes including elimination of cancer cells and virus infected cells. NK cells comprise a majority of large granular lymphocytes circulating in peripheral blood with a minority derived from T cell lineage.

HARDCOVER ISBN: 978-1-53612-999-1
RETAIL PRICE: $230

PROTHROMBIN COMPLEX CONCENTRATES: ADVANCES IN RESEARCH AND CLINICAL APPLICATIONS

EDITOR: Michael S. Firstenberg, M.D.

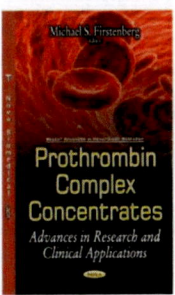

SERIES: Recent Advances in Hematology Research

BOOK DESCRIPTION: The goal of this book is to illustrate the spectrum of applications for prothrombin complex concentrates. The chapters trace the development of these agents, their mechanisms of action, the potential clinical applications, and highlight the key literature concerning their use.

HARDCOVER ISBN: 978-1-53610-694-7
RETAIL PRICE: $95

To see a complete list of Nova publications, please visit our website at www.novapublishers.com

Related Nova Publications

A Closer Look at Blood Serum

Editor: Josefine Boubacar

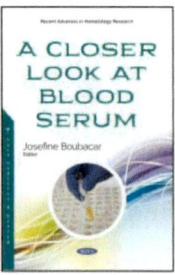

Series: Recent Advances in Hematology Research

Book Description: The opening chapter of this compilation is dedicated to the quantification of selenium and platinum in blood serum by electrothermal atomic absorption spectrometry.

Softcover ISBN: 978-1-53615-557-0
Retail Price: $82

Thrombotic Thrombocytopenic Purpura: Causes, Diagnosis and Treatment

Editor: Mason Hillam

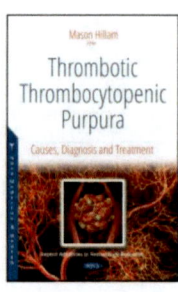

Series: Recent Advances in Hematology Research

Book Description: In the opening study included in *Thrombotic Thrombocytopenic Purpura: Causes, Diagnosis and Treatment,* the authors analyze the principal risk factors and causes of this disorder.

Softcover ISBN: 978-1-53615-353-8
Retail Price: $82

To see a complete list of Nova publications, please visit our website at www.novapublishers.com